Vaccine Safety Research, Data Access, AND Public Trust

Committee on the Review of the National Immunization Program's
Research Procedures and Data Sharing Program

Board on Health Promotion and Disease Prevention

INSTITUTE OF MEDICINE
OF THE NATIONAL ACADEMIES

THE NATIONAL ACADEMIES PRESS
Washington, D.C.
www.nap.edu

THE NATIONAL ACADEMIES PRESS 500 Fifth Street, N.W. Washington, DC 20001

NOTICE: The project that is the subject of this report was approved by the Governing Board of the National Research Council, whose members are drawn from the councils of the National Academy of Sciences, the National Academy of Engineering, and the Institute of Medicine. The members of the committee responsible for the report were chosen for their special competences and with regard for appropriate balance.

This study was supported by Contract No. 200-2000-00629, Task Order No. 23 between the National Academy of Sciences and the Centers for Disease Control and Prevention, U.S. Department of Health and Human Services. Any opinions, findings, conclusions, or recommendations expressed in this publication are those of the author(s) and do not necessarily reflect the view of the organizations or agencies that provided support for this project.

Library of Congress Cataloging-in-Publication Data

Institute of Medicine (U.S.). Committee on the Review of the National Immunization Program's Research Procedures and Data Sharing Program.
  Vaccine safety research, data access, and public trust / Committee on the Review of the National Immunization Program's Research Procedures and Data Sharing Program, Board on Health Promotion and Disease Prevention.
     p. ; cm.
  Includes bibliographical references.
  ISBN 0-309-09591-3 (pbk.) —ISBN 0-309-54874-8 (PDF)
  1. Vaccination—United States—Safety measures—Databases. 2. Vaccines—United States—Safety measures—Databases.
  [DNLM: 1. Vaccines—standards. 2. Access to Information. 3. Database Management Systems. 4. Public Opinion. 5. Safety—standards. 6. Trust—psychology. QW 805 I5914 2005] I. Title.
  RA638.I555 2005
  614.4'7—dc22   2005007271

Additional copies of this report are available from the National Academies Press, 500 Fifth Street, N.W., Lockbox 285, Washington, DC 20055; (800) 624-6242 or (202) 334-3313 (in the Washington metropolitan area); Internet, http://www.nap.edu.

For more information about the Institute of Medicine, visit the IOM home page at: **www.iom.edu**.

Copyright 2005 by the National Academy of Sciences. All rights reserved.

Printed in the United States of America.

The serpent has been a symbol of long life, healing, and knowledge among almost all cultures and religions since the beginning of recorded history. The serpent adopted as a logotype by the Institute of Medicine is a relief carving from ancient Greece, now held by the Staatliche Museen in Berlin.

*"Knowing is not enough; we must apply.
Willing is not enough; we must do."*
—Goethe

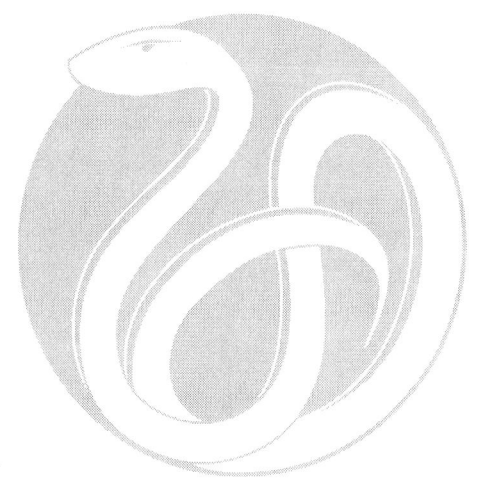

INSTITUTE OF MEDICINE
OF THE NATIONAL ACADEMIES

Adviser to the Nation to Improve Health

THE NATIONAL ACADEMIES
Advisers to the Nation on Science, Engineering, and Medicine

The **National Academy of Sciences** is a private, nonprofit, self-perpetuating society of distinguished scholars engaged in scientific and engineering research, dedicated to the furtherance of science and technology and to their use for the general welfare. Upon the authority of the charter granted to it by the Congress in 1863, the Academy has a mandate that requires it to advise the federal government on scientific and technical matters. Dr. Bruce M. Alberts is president of the National Academy of Sciences.

The **National Academy of Engineering** was established in 1964, under the charter of the National Academy of Sciences, as a parallel organization of outstanding engineers. It is autonomous in its administration and in the selection of its members, sharing with the National Academy of Sciences the responsibility for advising the federal government. The National Academy of Engineering also sponsors engineering programs aimed at meeting national needs, encourages education and research, and recognizes the superior achievements of engineers. Dr. Wm. A. Wulf is president of the National Academy of Engineering.

The **Institute of Medicine** was established in 1970 by the National Academy of Sciences to secure the services of eminent members of appropriate professions in the examination of policy matters pertaining to the health of the public. The Institute acts under the responsibility given to the National Academy of Sciences by its congressional charter to be an adviser to the federal government and, upon its own initiative, to identify issues of medical care, research, and education. Dr. Harvey V. Fineberg is president of the Institute of Medicine.

The **National Research Council** was organized by the National Academy of Sciences in 1916 to associate the broad community of science and technology with the Academy's purposes of furthering knowledge and advising the federal government. Functioning in accordance with general policies determined by the Academy, the Council has become the principal operating agency of both the National Academy of Sciences and the National Academy of Engineering in providing services to the government, the public, and the scientific and engineering communities. The Council is administered jointly by both Academies and the Institute of Medicine. Dr. Bruce M. Alberts and Dr. Wm. A. Wulf are chair and vice chair, respectively, of the National Research Council.

www.national-academies.org

COMMITTEE ON THE REVIEW OF THE NATIONAL IMMUNIZATION PROGRAM'S RESEARCH PROCEDURES AND DATA SHARING PROGRAM

JOHN C. BAILAR III M.D., Ph.D. (*Chair*), Professor Emeritus, University of Chicago, Washington, DC
GARNET L. ANDERSON, Ph.D., Co-Principal Investigator, Women's Health Initiative Clinical Coordinating Center, Fred Hutchinson Cancer Research Center, Seattle, WA
STEPHEN E. FIENBERG, Ph.D., Maurice Falk University Professor of Statistics and Social Science, Carnegie Mellon University, Pittsburgh, PA
DEBRA R. LAPPIN, J.D., Senior Advisor, B&D Sagamore, Public Health and Life Sciences Consulting, Washington, DC
MYRON M. LEVINE, M.D., D.T.P.H., Professor and Director, Center for Vaccine Development, School of Medicine, University of Maryland at Baltimore
ANNA C. MASTROIANNI, J.D., M.P.H., Assistant Professor, School of Law and Institute for Public Health Genetics, University of Washington, Seattle
COLIN L. SOSKOLNE, Ph.D., Professor, Department of Public Health Sciences, University of Alberta, Edmonton, Canada
ELAINE VAUGHAN, Ph.D., Associate Professor, Department of Psychology and Social Behavior, School of Social Ecology, University of California, Irvine

Study Staff

ANDREA PERNACK ANASON, M.P.H., Study Director
AMY GROSSMAN, Research Associate
RUTH KANTHULA, Senior Program Assistant
NORMAN GROSSBLATT, ELS (D), Senior Editor
ROSE MARIE MARTINEZ, Sc.D., Director, Board on Health Promotion and Disease Prevention

Reviewers

This report has been reviewed in draft form by individuals chosen for their diverse perspectives and technical expertise, in accordance with procedures approved by the National Research Council's (NRC's) Report Review Committee. The purpose of this independent review is to provide candid and critical comments that will assist the institution in making its published report as sound as possible and to ensure that the report meets institutional standards for objectivity, evidence, and responsiveness to the study charge. The review comments and draft manuscript remain confidential to protect the integrity of the deliberative process. We wish to thank the following individuals for their review of this report:

Alfred Berg, University of Washington, Seattle
Ann Bostrom, Georgia Institute of Technology, Atlanta
Alan Karr, National Institute of Statistical Sciences, Research Triangle Park, NC
Kristin Nichol, University of Minnesota, Minneapolis
Sarah Putney, Harvard University, Boston, MA
Jonathan Samet, Johns Hopkins University, Baltimore, MD
Brian Strom, University of Pennsylvania, Philadelphia
Frances Visco, National Breast Cancer Coalition, Washington, DC
Robert Woolson, Medical University of South Carolina, Charleston

Although the reviewers listed above have provided many constructive comments and suggestions, they were not asked to endorse the conclusions or recommendations nor did they see the final draft of the report before its release. The review of this report was overseen by **Neal A. Vanselow**, Tulane University, and **Joseph P. Newhouse**, Harvard University. Appointed by the NRC and Institute of Medicine, they were responsible for making certain that an independent examination of this report was carried out in accordance with institutional procedures and that all review comments were carefully considered. Responsibility for the final content of this report rests entirely with the authoring committee and the institution.

Contents

EXECUTIVE SUMMARY   1

1 STUDY BACKGROUND AND CONTEXTUAL ISSUES   13
Charge to the Committee, 14
Study Process, 16
Context of This Study, 17
Issues Framing the Committee's Deliberations, 19
Previous Release of Preliminary Findings from the Vaccine
   Safety Datalink, 20
How Trust Affects the Vaccine Safety Datalink, 21
Overarching Principles, 23

2 DESCRIPTION OF THE VACCINE SAFETY DATALINK   25
Role of FDA and CDC in Assessing Vaccine Safety, 25
Development of the Vaccine Safety Datalink, 28
Complexity and Limitations of the Vaccine Safety Datalink
   Database, 29
The Shelby Amendment and the Information Quality Act, 31

3 THE VACCINE SAFETY DATALINK DATA
SHARING PROGRAM   33
Design and Implementation to Date of the Vaccine Safety
   Datalink Data Sharing Program, 33
The Vaccine Safety Datalink Data Sharing Program's Ability to
   Share Data, 35

Current Standards of Practice of Similar Data Sharing Programs, 37
Framework of Recommendations on Access to Vaccine
   Safety Datalink Data, 58
Limitations of Data Available Through the Vaccine Safety
   Datalink Data Sharing Program, 59
Specific Components of the Vaccine Safety Datalink Data
   Sharing Program Guidelines, 65

4 THE VACCINE SAFETY DATALINK RESEARCH PROCESS
   AND THE RELEASE OF PRELIMINARY FINDINGS   76
   Review of Iterative Analysis Approaches Used for
      Vaccine Safety Datalink Studies, 76
   Vaccine Safety Datalink Research Plan, 80
   Sharing Vaccine Safety Datalink Program Information, 83
   The Role of Peer Review, 85
   Release of Preliminary Findings, 87

5 INDEPENDENT REVIEW OF VACCINE SAFETY
   DATALINK ACTIVITIES   96
   NVAC Subcommittee to Review and Provide Advice on
      the Vaccine Safety Datalink Research Plan, 97
   Independent Committee to Review Vaccine Safety Datalink
      Research Proposals and Provide Advice on the Release of
      Preliminary Findings, 99

CONCLUDING REMARKS   104

REFERENCES   105

APPENDIXES

A Committee Biographies   111
B Glossary   115
C Acronyms   117
D Meeting One—Agenda   119
E Meeting Two—Agenda   123
F Summary of Public Submissions   127
G Notice and Request for Comment on *Procedures and Costs
   for Use of the Research Data Center*   132

Executive Summary

BACKGROUND

The Vaccine Safety Datalink (VSD) is a large linked database that was created in 1991 to fill a void in the ability of the United States to study vaccine safety issues. The VSD was developed through the collaborative efforts of the National Immunization Program (NIP) at the Centers for Disease Control and Prevention (CDC) and several private managed care organizations (MCOs) (Chen et al., 1997). The VSD is a unique national resource for evaluating vaccine safety. It includes data from administrative records for more than 7 million members of eight MCOs (Davis, 2004). The VSD database links data on patient characteristics, health outcomes (according to data resulting from inpatient, outpatient, and emergency-room records), and vaccination history (vaccine type, date of vaccination, manufacturer, lot number, and injection site) (Davis, 2004). The VSD can be a valuable tool for the retrospective assessment of vaccine safety because the number of people included is large, they generally receive most of their health services at the MCOs, and demographic, health outcome, and vaccination data are maintained electronically.

The opportunities offered by the VSD for thorough investigations of vaccine safety concerns and well-designed, planned, retrospective vaccine studies have led to heightened interest in the results of VSD studies and sometimes in the VSD data themselves. A few researchers interested in particular vaccine safety hypotheses also have shown interest in accessing and analyzing VSD data. The interest in the VSD shown by researchers, advocacy groups, members of Congress, and others has brought increasing attention to its use, its limitations, and the implications of studies that were conducted through the analysis of its data.

Throughout the first decade of the VSD's existence, researchers from the NIP and the MCOs participating in the VSD collaborated on studies that used VSD data. During that time, there was no way for an independent external researcher who did not pursue a collaborative relationship with a NIP-affiliated or MCO-affiliated researcher to use the VSD. In 2002, after requests by independent external researchers that VSD data be made available, the NIP announced the creation of the VSD data sharing program (CDC, 2004d). The VSD data sharing program guidelines (CDC, 2002, 2003a, 2004a,b,c) have been revised multiple times since the inception of the program.

Concerns about data sharing were stimulated in part by public concern over a study initiated in 1999 using VSD data. In fall 1999, researchers at the NIP began a screening study using VSD data to investigate whether exposure to thimerosal in vaccines (to which it was added as a preservative) was associated with neurodevelopmental disorders (DeStefano, 2004; Verstraeten et al., 2003a). Some members of the general public have criticized the thimerosal screening study for changes in the original study protocol, changes in eligibility criteria, the selective official release of preliminary findings, and the inclusion of vaccine-manufacturer representatives in a meeting intended to provide external expert review of the study (Bernard, 2004).

CHARGE TO THE COMMITTEE

The Institute of Medicine Committee on the Review of the National Immunization Program's Research Procedures and Data Sharing Program was asked to address the following charge:[1]

(1a) review the design and the implementation to date of the new Vaccine Safety Datalink Data Sharing Program to assess compliance with the current standards of practice for data sharing in the scientific community and (1b) make recommendations to the National Immunization Program and the National Center for Health Statistics for any needed modifications that would facilitate use, ensure appropriate utilization, and protect confidentiality; and (2a) review the iterative approaches to conducting analysis that are characteristics of studies using the complex, automated

---

[1] After the transfer of some administrative responsibilities for the VSD from the NIP to the National Center for Health Statistics, the charge was modified on August 31, 2004, to include "and the National Center for Health Statistics" in section 1b of the charge. The charge was modified on November 17, 2004, to substitute "preliminary findings" for "preliminary data" in sections 2b and 2c.

Vaccine Safety Datalink system. Examples of recent studies to be examined are a completed screening study on thimerosal and vaccines (Verstraeten et al.) and cohort studies on asthma; (2b) review whether, when, and how preliminary findings about potential vaccine-related risks obtained from the Vaccine Safety Datalink system should be shared with other scientists, communicated to the public, and used to make policy or recommendations to CDC; and (2c) make recommendations to the National Immunization Program on the release of such preliminary findings in the future.

The charge was expanded to include the National Center for Health Statistics (NCHS) in part 1 because organizational responsibility for the VSD data sharing program was transferred from the NIP to NCHS in March 2004.

OVERARCHING PRINCIPLES

In the course of its deliberations, the committee found that several overarching principles emerged. The principles can be described as common themes inherent in the committee's recommendations and thus principles that should be considered in any modifications of the VSD data sharing program or any determinations about whether, when, and how to release VSD preliminary findings. The four overarching principles that emerged from the committee's recommendations are these:

- *Independence*. Ensure that potential biases and potential conflicts of interest are minimized, balanced, or otherwise managed in the design and implementation of all processes, practices, and policies related to the VSD.
- *Transparency*. Ensure that all processes, practices, and policies related to the VSD are developed in the spirit of openness, clearly articulated, and easily available to interested persons or entities, and that any deviations from them are documented and justified.
- *Fairness*. Ensure that all processes, practices, and policies related to the VSD are designed and implemented in a fair manner.
- *Protection of confidentiality*. Ensure that the design and implementation of the VSD protect the confidentiality of individually identifiable information.

CONTEXTUAL ISSUES

Concerns about trust and how the public perceives the reliability of findings based on VSD data have spilled over from the NIP's analyses to the development and implementation of the VSD data sharing program. Taking steps to improve the independence, transparency, and fairness of VSD procedures while continuing to protect confidentiality will help to enhance trust in the processes and procedures used for VSD research and the VSD data sharing program. Trust can be enhanced only if the public has confidence in the independence and fairness of the decision-making process for VSD research priorities and approval of VSD data sharing proposals.

The VSD is a public resource that is designed to inform important public health policy decisions. Though it is a resource supported by public funds, there are restrictions on access because the data are provided by and remain the property of private MCOs. By the very nature of its potential to influence policy, the public demands and deserves access to the data used to influence those decisions and transparency in the processes that permit or restrict access. If the VSD is intended to be used as a foundation of policy decisions, there is a public need to share data fairly and to be as transparent as possible while protecting the confidentiality of individually identifiable information in the VSD. Confidentiality protections must not be jeopardized; a single breach of confidentiality, no matter how minor, could undermine the contractual arrangements between the MCOs and the NIP and lead to the termination of cooperation and the loss of a unique resource of potentially great national value.

The committee determined that it could not adequately address issues of independence, transparency, fairness, and protection of confidentiality without examining how the VSD research process supports or hinders the application of those principles. When concerns arise about the independence and transparency, in particular, of the general VSD research process, those concerns spill over to people's perception of the independence and transparency of the VSD data sharing program and of the determinations about whether, when, and how to release VSD preliminary findings. To provide the most appropriate and useful recommendations requested in its charge, the committee believed that it had to consider how the VSD research plan, the priority-setting of VSD studies, and the VSD peer-review process affect the VSD data sharing program and the release of preliminary findings.

The committee's recommendations are related to four main topics: the VSD data sharing program; the release of preliminary findings based on VSD data; independent review of VSD activities; and the applicability of the Shelby Amendment and Information Quality Act to VSD data and VSD preliminary findings.

THE VACCINE SAFETY DATALINK DATA SHARING PROGRAM

Reflecting on all the information gathered throughout its study, the committee finds that the VSD data sharing program has three short-term goals:

EXECUTIVE SUMMARY

1. To facilitate access to and use of the VSD;
2. To protect the confidentiality of individually identifiable data in the VSD; and
3. To enhance public trust in the VSD as a tool to address specific concerns about vaccine safety.

On the basis of those three goals, the committee developed its recommendations related to the VSD data sharing program in the following framework:

- The NIP should support the broadest feasible use of the VSD for vaccine safety research within the constraints of law, protection of confidentiality, and VSD contract provisions;
- Bureaucratic and technical barriers to accessing the VSD should be minimized, although some types of studies may require collaboration with or facilitation by data custodians;
- Guidelines for proposals from independent external researchers should be developed and publicized to facilitate access;
- Responses to proposals should be timely;
- Criteria for the independent review of proposals should be publicly accessible;
- Costs to researchers should approximate the incremental costs of access;
- Descriptions of the objectives and methods of current and published studies should be made publicly available;
- All VSD users should provide a timely and detailed public report of their results to the NIP; and
- All completed VSD studies should be subjected to scientific peer review before any public release.

LIMITATIONS OF THE VACCINE SAFETY DATALINK DATA SHARING PROGRAM AND THE NEED FOR COLLABORATION

The VSD and the VSD data sharing program have a number of limitations. Because VSD data come from administrative databases of the MCOs, additional data collection (for example, medical-chart reviews) or data cleaning must be done before the automated data are suitable for many specific research studies. For new vaccine safety studies, the VSD data sharing program allows external researchers access only to automated data and only to data from before 2001 (CDC, 2004a). Because the quality of automated data cannot be guaranteed, the inclusion of chart-review-verified data in new vaccine safety studies improves the quality of such studies. Chart-review-verified data can be obtained only by collaborating with NIP-affiliated or MCO-affiliated researchers. Thus, it is important for independent external researchers to try to collaborate with a NIP-affiliated or MCO-affiliated researcher to produce a new, high-quality vaccine safety study with VSD data from 2001 and later.

Because of the limitations of the data available through the program and the differing levels of access to VSD data that depend on the type of researcher requesting access, the VSD data sharing program does not meet the traditional definition of data sharing. For the VSD data sharing program to be considered a true data sharing program, changes must be made.

All the committee's recommendations related to the VSD data sharing program can be found in Box ES-1 at the end of this executive summary.

RELEASE OF PRELIMINARY FINDINGS BASED ON VACCINE SAFETY DATALINK DATA

Solely internal peer-review processes may be needed when preliminary findings could have a substantial impact on public health. The need to release preliminary findings rapidly may force a decision to limit peer review to peers inside the federal government, but if so, the internal peer review should be as extensive as possible. In such situations, purely internal review should be followed by external review on an expedited schedule. In the case of the VSD, however, the committee finds that because the data are incorporated into the VSD data files annually rather than continually, there will rarely be situations in which preliminary findings are so urgent that they cannot undergo independent external peer review.

Numerous concerns arise in the release of preliminary findings, but in some situations it is appropriate to release preliminary findings about potential vaccine-related risks. Conditions governing whether, when, and how to share preliminary VSD findings with other scientists, the public, and policy-makers should be defined a priori. Release of preliminary findings shared with others, used to make policy decisions, or superseded by later findings are special situations that require special considerations. Any preliminary findings that are released under such conditions need to be communicated in an appropriate context.

All the committee's recommendations related to the release of preliminary findings based on VSD data can be found in Box ES-1 at the end of this executive summary.

INDEPENDENT REVIEW OF VACCINE SAFETY DATALINK ACTIVITIES

There are legitimate concerns about the independence and fairness of the implementation of review procedures applied to VSD data sharing proposals and of determinations about the release of preliminary findings from VSD analyses. The lack of transparency of some of the processes also affects the trust relationship between the NIP and the general public. To address some of those concerns, the committee recommends that two independent groups be used.

To give the full array of stakeholders an opportunity to provide input into the VSD research plan priority-setting process and to ensure that the process is as transparent as possible, an independent group should be used to review and provide advice on the VSD research plan. **The committee recommends that a subcommittee of the National Vaccine Advisory Committee that includes representatives of a wide variety of stakeholders (such as advocacy groups, vaccine manufacturers, FDA, and CDC) review and provide advice to the NIP on the VSD research plan annually. The subcommittee charged with this role could be the existing Subcommittee on Safety and Communications or a subcommittee created specifically for the purpose.**

In addition, to enhance trust in the fairness of the VSD research process, an independent review committee (advisory to the director of CDC) with minimal and balanced biases and conflicts of interest should be established to review various aspects of VSD research activities and of the VSD data sharing program. **The committee recommends that an independent review committee with minimal and balanced biases and conflicts of interest be created to:**

- **Review independent external researchers' proposals to use VSD data through the data sharing program;**
- **Review research proposals from internal researchers and provide oversight of changes in or deviations from research protocols for internal VSD studies; and**
- **Provide advice on when and how preliminary findings based on VSD data should be made public.**

The committee makes other recommendations throughout its report that focus on specific issues related to the VSD data sharing program and the determination of whether, when, and how to release preliminary findings. However, the committee's recommendations regarding independent oversight of VSD-related activities are the primary means of improving transparency and ensuring fair implementation of processes, practices, and policies related to VSD access, and thereby enhancing public trust in the use of the VSD to answer vaccine safety questions.

CONCLUDING REMARKS

The VSD database has many strengths, but it also has limitations. The value of the VSD data sharing program will be enhanced by easy access to the data, so that a variety of researchers can conduct a range of studies and have their findings reviewed by peers and discussed in ways conducive to the advancement of knowledge about vaccine safety. The VSD is a valuable resource for the nation. Efforts should be made to facilitate access to VSD data and their appropriate utilization, while protecting the confidentiality of information contained therein. Ensuring the independence, transparency, and fairness of VSD research activities is important for ensuring public trust in the VSD as a tool for addressing critical vaccine safety questions.

BOX ES-1
Committee Recommendations

Chapter 2:
DESCRIPTION OF THE VACCINE SAFETY DATALINK

Recommendation 2.1: The committee recommends that the NIP and NCHS seek legal advice to clarify the applicability of the Shelby Amendment and the Information Quality Act to VSD data and VSD preliminary findings.

Chapter 3:
THE VACCINE SAFETY DATALINK DATA SHARING PROGRAM

Recommendation 3.1: The committee recommends that future revisions of the VSD data sharing guidelines clearly and explicitly describe the VSD data that are and are not available to independent external researchers for new vaccine studies through the VSD data sharing program.

Recommendation 3.2: The committee recommends that the distinction between the annual automated VSD data (whose quality cannot always be guaranteed) available to independent external researchers through the data sharing program and the study-specific data potentially available to researchers affiliated with the NIP or the participating MCOs be explained more clearly in the data sharing guidelines so that potential users are informed about the limitations of the data that are available through the data sharing program.

EXECUTIVE SUMMARY 9

BOX ES-1 Continued

Recommendation 3.3: Because of the limitations in the data available to independent external researchers through the VSD data sharing program, the committee recommends that the NIP require the designation of a facilitator for collaboration at each MCO as a condition of the VSD contract.

Recommendation 3.4: To formulate alternative hypotheses or to conduct alternative analyses, researchers need to have access to information or variables that would allow the use of different inclusion and exclusion criteria, different variables for inclusion in models, and, in general, earlier versions of a dataset that would support such restructuring. The committee believes that it is appropriate to allow independent external researchers access to such datasets and recommends that such datasets be made available through the VSD data sharing program.

Recommendation 3.5: The committee recommends that the VSD data sharing guidelines reflect a more specific categorization of the types of studies that can be done with VSD data to conceptualize the full range of studies that independent external researchers may wish to conduct with the data: an audit, a broader reanalysis, a corroboration study, and an investigation of a new hypothesis.

Recommendation 3.6: The committee recommends that there be specific evaluation criteria for VSD proposals and that interested persons have an opportunity to comment on the draft evaluation criteria before they are finalized; the evaluation criteria should be identified clearly in the VSD data sharing guidelines.

Recommendation 3.7: The committee recommends that the technical feasibility of a proposed VSD study be the primary evaluation criterion in the review of proposals submitted to the VSD data sharing program.

Recommendation 3.8: To assist independent external researchers who want to use VSD data through the data sharing program, the committee recommends that the NIP and NCHS add to the VSD data sharing program guidelines a list of recommended competencies for VSD data analysis.

Recommendation 3.9: To facilitate use of the VSD data sharing program, the committee recommends that the NIP work with the VSD-participating MCOs to determine the feasibility of using IRB authorization agreements for VSD research proposals.

Recommendation 3.10: The committee recommends that the NIP work with the MCOs participating in the VSD and America's Health Insurance Plans (the VSD contractor) to evaluate the feasibility of streamlining the

Continued

BOX ES-1 Continued

IRB review process for audits or broader reanalyses in accordance with appropriate regulations.

Recommendation 3.11: Because the confidentiality concerns are integral to the continuation of the VSD, the committee recommends that NCHS in conjunction with the MCOs develop policies and procedures to address confidentiality violations of VSD data and that they be clearly described in the VSD data sharing program guidelines and the agreements that external researchers must sign before using the RDC.

Recommendation 3.12: The committee concludes that it is reasonable to expect researchers who request access to VSD data to have their own funding and it therefore recommends that RDC costs not be waived for independent external researchers.

Recommendation 3.13: The committee recommends that, as a condition of accessing VSD data, all independent external researchers that use the VSD data sharing program be required to submit a report to the NIP (with a copy to NCHS) within a reasonable time (to be determined by the NIP) on the status of their study, the type of study conducted (an audit, a broader reanalysis, a corroboration study, or an investigation of a new hypothesis), the results obtained, and their planned further activities. The reports should be made public by the NIP and should be easily accessible.

Recommendation 3.14: The committee recommends that, as a condition of accessing VSD data, all independent external researchers that use the VSD data sharing program be required to submit to the NIP (with a copy to NCHS) a copy of a manuscript intended for publication at least 30 days before submission to a journal or other print or electronic media. Copies of presentations to be delivered at conferences or meetings that are open to the public or that have media coverage should also be submitted to the NIP and NCHS at least 15 days before presentation.

Chapter 4:
THE VACCINE SAFETY DATALINK RESEARCH PROCESS AND THE RELEASE OF PRELIMINARY FINDINGS

Recommendation 4.1: To enhance the value of the VSD, to improve the credibility of results derived from it, and to support CDC's role in assessing vaccine safety, the committee recommends that the NIP develop an annual VSD research plan. The plan should define the priorities for new studies and support of current studies. The annual VSD research plan should be made public. Material deviations from the plan should be identified and be publicly available.

BOX ES-1 Continued

Recommendation 4.2: To support greater use of the VSD and to promote opportunities for collaborative work outside the existing community of VSD researchers, the committee recommends that the annual VSD research plan include provisions for allocating some existing funds, on a competitive basis, to external researchers interested in conducting collaborative work with VSD data.

Recommendation 4.3: The committee recommends that detailed research protocols for each study conducted by an internal VSD researcher be developed, peer-reviewed, and archived. Each protocol should include well-specified definitions of the study population, exposures, and cases; detailed analytic plans; sample size requirements; and study timelines. Data collection forms, procedures, data and analysis files, programming code, and database versions should be documented, cataloged, and archived for a period of at least 7 years after completion of a study.

Recommendation 4.4: To promote collaboration and information-sharing, the committee recommends that the NIP update and improve its list of publications and presentations by establishing a VSD research clearinghouse that provides on a timely basis status reports, study findings, and conclusions for current and completed VSD studies.

Recommendation 4.5: The committee recommends that the NIP and NCHS release publicly the procedures that will be used for record-keeping of VSD data sharing program documents and update the status of the program regularly.

Recommendation 4.6: The committee recommends that in nearly all situations preliminary findings from the VSD be subject to independent external peer review before being communicated to the public or used as the basis of a policy decision. When CDC determines that purely internal peer review is necessary before release, external peer review should be undertaken as soon as possible.

Recommendation 4.7: The committee recommends that preliminary findings from VSD data be shared with the public whenever the findings are presented to anyone other than collaborators in the research, federal employees responsible for research activities, MCO-affiliated VSD researchers, scientific journals, peer reviewers for scientific journals, and people responsible for oversight of the research.

Recommendation 4.8: The committee recommends that preliminary findings from VSD data be shared with the public whenever these findings contribute to the basis of a policy decision or are used to change guidelines on vaccine administration.

Continued

BOX ES-1 Continued

Recommendation 4.9: The committee recommends that when final results from VSD analyses or studies are released through publication or through presentation at a meeting, preliminary findings be shared only rarely, but that the dataset from which the final results were obtained be available to other researchers who may verify and extend the results through an audit or broader reanalysis.

Recommendation 4.10: The committee recommends that any preliminary findings based on VSD data that are shared with the public be put into appropriate statistical and scientific context with clear characterization of the uncertainties in the findings, of the strengths and limitations of the data, and of the possibility that new data or new analyses could change interpretations.

Chapter 5:
INDEPENDENT REVIEW OF VACCINE SAFETY DATALINK ACTIVITIES

Recommendation 5.1: The committee recommends that a subcommittee of the National Vaccine Advisory Committee that includes representatives of a wide variety of stakeholders (such as advocacy groups, vaccine manufacturers, FDA, and CDC) review and provide advice to the NIP on the VSD research plan annually. The subcommittee charged with this role could be the existing Subcommittee on Safety and Communications or a subcommittee created specifically for the purpose.

Recommendation 5.2: The committee recommends that the NIP propose to the National Vaccine Program that additional liaison representatives be appointed to ensure that all perspectives are heard by adequately representing advocacy groups and other members of the public at subcommittee meetings addressing the VSD research plan.

Recommendation 5.3: The committee recommends that an independent review committee with minimal and balanced biases and conflicts of interest be created to:
- Review independent external researchers' proposals to use VSD data through the data sharing program;
- Review research proposals from internal researchers and provide oversight of changes in or deviations from research protocols for internal VSD studies; and
- Provide advice on when and how preliminary findings based on VSD data should be made public.

1

Study Background and Contextual Issues

Vaccines are regarded as among the greatest public health achievements of the twentieth century (CDC, 1999a). Their use has drastically reduced morbidity and mortality from infectious diseases throughout the world. Indeed, most people in industrialized countries now have little or no recollection of epidemics of polio or smallpox or of the occurrence of pertussis. However, although incidences of vaccine-preventable infectious diseases continue to be very low in the United States, there is always a risk that low population vaccination rates will contribute to outbreaks of infectious diseases that previously were held at bay (such as recent measles and pertussis outbreaks in the United Kingdom and the United States) (CDC, 1993; Jansen et al., 2003).

The current extremely low incidences of many childhood infectious diseases (such as polio, mumps, and rubella) and thus the low risk of long-term damage or death from these diseases in the United States and other industrialized countries have led to detailed studies of the risk-benefit balance of vaccines. In 1971, for example, concerns about the well-documented frequency of adverse reactions to the smallpox vaccine, the elimination of endemic smallpox in the Western Hemisphere, and the excellent progress made in the World Health Organization smallpox eradication program by that time led the U.S. government to suspend the routine vaccination of children against smallpox because the risk of adverse effects of the vaccine in children and their family contacts was deemed greater than the risk of the disease itself (CDC, 1971).

In the United States, the Department of Health and Human Services, through the Food and Drug Administration (FDA) and the Centers for Disease Control and Prevention (CDC), has responsibility for ensuring vaccine safety. Within CDC, the National Immunization Program (NIP) is responsible for assisting health departments with immunization programs, supporting the establishment of vaccine supply contracts, administering research and operational programs for the prevention and control of vaccine-preventable diseases, and monitoring the safety and efficacy of vaccines (CDC, 2001). The NIP, in conjunction with its colleagues at FDA, uses a variety of means to continually evaluate vaccine safety, including signal detection through reports from the Vaccine Adverse Event Reporting System (VAERS), ad hoc epidemiologic studies, state and community immunization registries, and laboratory surveillance. Another resource that has been used since 1991 to evaluate vaccine safety is the Vaccine Safety Datalink (VSD).

The VSD is a large linked database that was developed in 1991 through the collaborative efforts of CDC and several private managed care organizations (MCOs) (Chen et al., 1997). The VSD currently includes data from administrative records for more than 7 million members of eight MCOs (Davis, 2004). In the VSD, vaccination records, patient characteristics, and health outcomes are linked; this allows the VSD to serve as a unique and potentially powerful resource for the ongoing evaluation of vaccine safety (Davis, 2004). With its longitudinal data on reasonably well-defined cohorts, the VSD differs from VAERS, a passive surveillance system that depends on voluntary reporting. Both data sources have strengths and limitations, but they complement one another.

The opportunities offered by the VSD for thorough investigations of vaccine safety concerns and well-designed, planned, retrospective vaccine studies have led to heightened interest in the results of VSD studies and sometimes in the VSD data themselves. A few researchers interested in particular vaccine safety hypotheses also have shown interest in accessing and analyzing VSD data. The interest in the VSD shown by researchers, advocacy groups, members of Congress, and others has brought increasing attention to its use, its limitations, and the implications of studies that were conducted through the analysis of its data.

CHARGE TO THE COMMITTEE

The Institute of Medicine (IOM) Committee on the Review of the National Immunization Program's Research Procedures and Data Sharing Program was convened at the request of the NIP to offer advice on two

STUDY BACKGROUND AND CONTEXTUAL ISSUES

issues related to the VSD. The NIP asked IOM to convene a panel of experts to address the following charge:[1]

> (1a) review the design and the implementation to date of the new Vaccine Safety Datalink Data Sharing Program to assess compliance with the current standards of practice for data sharing in the scientific community and, (1b) make recommendations to the National Immunization Program and the National Center for Health Statistics for any needed modifications that would facilitate use, ensure appropriate utilization, and protect confidentiality and (2a) review the iterative approaches to conducting analysis that are characteristics of studies using the complex, automated Vaccine Safety Datalink system. Examples of recent studies to be examined are a completed screening study on thimerosal and vaccines (Verstraeten et al.) and cohort studies on asthma; (2b) review whether, when, and how preliminary findings about potential vaccine-related risks obtained from the Vaccine Safety Datalink system should be shared with other scientists, communicated to the public, and used to make policy or recommendations to CDC; and (2c) make recommendations to the National Immunization Program on the release of such preliminary findings in the future.

The charge was expanded to include the National Center for Health Statistics (NCHS) in part 1 of the charge because organizational responsibility for the VSD data sharing program was transferred from the NIP to NCHS in March 2004. The recommendations related to the VSD data sharing program apply to both the NIP and NCHS; the recommendations related to the release of preliminary findings apply to only the NIP.

In response to the NIP request, the IOM assembled a committee of experts in epidemiology, biostatistics, research design, research ethics, vaccine research, risk communication, and public input into the scientific process. (See Appendix A for committee biographies.) This report is the committee's response to the charge.

Readers familiar with vaccine safety issues may be aware of the work of earlier IOM committees focused on vaccine safety. The Committee on the Review of the National Immunization Program's Research Procedures and Data Sharing Program is separate and distinct from other IOM committees. It was convened solely to address the charge stated above, and it has examined issues of process related to the VSD, not issues of scientific validity pertaining to specific VSD studies.

---

[1] After the transfer of some administrative responsibilities for the VSD from the NIP to the National Center for Health Statistics, the charge was modified on August 31, 2004, to include "and the National Center for Health Statistics" in section 1b of the charge. The charge was modified on November 17, 2004 to substitute "preliminary findings" for "preliminary data" in sections 2b and 2c.

STUDY PROCESS

The committee gathered information to address its charge through a variety of means. It held two information-gathering meetings that were open to the public. The first, on August 23-24, 2004, focused on the first part of its charge, the VSD data sharing program; its full agenda is in Appendix D. The second meeting, on October 21-22, 2004, focused on the second part of the committee's charge, the release of preliminary findings from the VSD; its full agenda is in Appendix E. The committee also held a closed meeting on December 13-14, 2004.

Each of the open meetings included a session for comments from the public, and many persons did speak. Both meetings were Webcast in real time so that members of the public could listen to the proceedings and send questions to the committee by e-mail. The committee also received public submissions of material for its consideration at the meetings and by mail, e-mail, and fax throughout the course of the study. A list of the public submissions received by the committee is in Appendix F.

A Web site (http://www.iom.edu/nipdatasharing) and a listserv were created to provide information to the public about the committee's work and to facilitate communication with the committee. Many of the speakers' presentation slides from the two information-gathering meetings are available in electronic format on the project's Web site.

Committee members and staff made informal visits to the NIP, NCHS, and one of the MCOs contributing data to the VSD to gain a greater understanding of the background and daily operations of the VSD data sharing program. The site visits provided additional background information for the committee. The committee developed a list of questions for the NIP and NCHS (submitted to the agencies after the August 23-24, 2004, committee meeting) that provided the context for the visits; the NIP and NCHS submitted a formal response to the committee's list of questions (CDC, 2004d).

A list of materials reviewed by the committee (in the form in which they were reviewed), including all submissions of information from the public and many items not cited in this report, can be obtained from the National Academies Public Access Records Office at (202)334-3543 or http://www.national-academies.org/publicaccess.

When the committee was convened, the NIP asked it to produce two reports—one on each part of the charge. In the course of its deliberations, however, the committee found that the two parts of its charge overlapped substantially. It concluded that it could provide its best advice to the NIP and NCHS if it thought broadly about solutions that would address all the overlapping concerns and if it integrated its findings, conclusions, and recommendations into a single report. It sought to recommend the best

STUDY BACKGROUND AND CONTEXTUAL ISSUES   17

solutions for issues inherent in the full charge; it would not have been able to provide its best advice if it viewed the two parts of the charge separately. The NIP permitted the committee to provide a single report, and this report thus responds to the committee's full charge.

CONTEXT OF THIS STUDY

To appreciate important elements of the societal context of this report, it is important to acknowledge the breadth and depth of concerns that are peripheral to this IOM study but related to the VSD. Concerns about public access to data, transparency of research activities, researchers' conflicts of interest, and confidentiality of individuals' information are an important part of the context of this study. The confluence of the concerns affects how the public, advocacy groups, researchers, the federal government, and MCOs approach vaccine safety and data sharing issues.

Over the last two decades, community engagement in the health enterprise generally and in vaccine safety activities in particular has come under increasing public scrutiny. Criticisms related to vaccine safety have been wide-ranging. Some people believe that the increase in the rate of autism is attributable to the use of thimerosal in vaccines (Fisher, 2004b; SafeMinds, 2004a), that CDC has used questionable research methods when examining that possibility (Bernard, 2004), that CDC is limiting access to the VSD to prevent the discovery of evidence about vaccine adverse reactions (Fisher, 2004b), and that oversight of vaccine safety activities should not be in the same CDC office that is responsible for promoting immunization (Copeland and Simpson, 2004; Fisher, 1999). NIP staff indicated to the committee that they have devoted much time to responding to those concerns (Bernier, 2004a). With greater attention to access to and use of VSD data, the MCOs participating in the VSD have indicated that they have spent considerable time on ensuring that proper procedures are in place to protect the confidentiality of VSD data (Wharton, 2004). Previous IOM committees that examined the evidence on particular vaccine safety questions also have been criticized by some groups (NVIC, 2004; SafeMinds, 2004b).

There has been increasing concern over the last few years about protecting the confidentiality of personal data, whether held by the U.S. government or by the private sector, that meet the definition of *protected health information* (HHS, 2003a). The Health Insurance Portability and Accountability Act (HIPAA) created new standards for the protection of the confidentiality of data meeting the definition (Pub. L. No. 104-191 [1996]). In 2003, a privacy rule was issued by DHHS to implement HIPAA (HHS, 2003a). Organizations subject to the privacy rule must have standards in place to address the use and disclosure of health information on individuals ("covered entities"). They must also have standards to help people to understand their privacy rights and how their health information is used (HHS, 2003a). The year 2002 saw passage of the Confidential Information Protection and Statistical Efficiency Act (CIPSEA), which requires that information not be disclosed in an identifiable form for any nonstatistical purpose unless there is formal consent from the individual (Pub. L. No. 107-347 [2002]). CIPSEA was enacted to establish uniform confidentiality protections and promote statistical efficiency by authorizing limited data sharing (Title V Pub. L. No. 107-347 [2002]); when a federal agency collects data for statistical use only, it can protect the data, and they will be exempt from release under the Freedom of Information Act (FOIA).

The demand by consumers for more information about issues affecting their health and the health of their families is growing and evolving. As evidenced by the recent public outcries over the alleged withholding of pharmaceutical risk information by FDA and pharmaceutical manufacturers, consumers insist that there be more and more transparency in the research processes, practices, and policies that affect their health. Litigation may also be a motivating force for requesting access to data and for performing particular studies. This can be considered a new era of consumer advocacy and consumer access, and the institutions that historically have controlled health information are still determining how to respond to evolving consumer demands.

The study reported here occurred at a time of increased focus on the transparency of U.S. government-funded research activities, including open access to the published results of federal research, to research databases, and to the results of clinical trials. The Information Quality Act, enacted in December 2000, requires federal agencies to establish a process for ensuring the "quality, objectivity, utility, and integrity" of the data and information disseminated to the public by the federal government (Pub. L. No. 106-554 [2000]; Copeland and Simpson, 2004). The Shelby Amendment (Pub. L. No. 105-277 [1998]), enacted in October 1998, required all federal agencies to ensure that data resulting from a grant award be made available to the public through FOIA (Gough and Milloy, 2000; Phillips, 2002). Federal agencies also have instituted other measures to promote and standardize data release. For example, both CDC and the National Institutes of Health (NIH) recently released data sharing guidelines (CDC, 2003b; NIH, 2004a) outlining the processes whereby data should be shared with other researchers. On September 3, 2004, NIH released for public comment a proposal requiring that final peer-reviewed manuscripts containing results of NIH-funded research be available in a free, publicly accessible database (PubMed Central) 6 months after publication, or sooner if the publisher agrees (NIH, 2004b). On February 3, 2005, after receiving 6,000 public comments, NIH announced the new policy that calls on scientists to voluntarily release to the public manuscripts from research supported by NIH as soon as possible, and within 12 months of final publication (NIH, 2005b). There is increasing public demand for the registration of current clinical trials to foster full transparency of clinical-trial research results. It is in that environment that the committee conducted its review and the committee's report has been developed.

Some people have criticized the NIP for how the VSD data sharing program was developed and implemented, for the processes used to conduct a thimerosal screening study (Verstraeten et al., 2003a), and for how the findings from that study were released and shared with interested stakeholders. The committee heard many of those concerns during the public comment periods at its two meetings and duly noted the level of concern expressed by many of the attendees, some of whom stated their frustration with the systems and processes in place for VSD data sharing. Many of the same sentiments were expressed in e-mails to the committee.

The committee has reviewed and considered all documents and other information submitted by the NIP, NCHS, independent external researchers, other groups, and the public, and it appreciates the thoughtful comments it has received. The committee has addressed its charge by deliberating the relevant issues with an ear open to the voices of all interested parties. The committee's report is not intended to resolve many of the specific points of contention around vaccine safety issues, but the processes for data sharing suggested by the committee should offer opportunities for greater public transparency and information sharing and consequently a means to address criticisms and enhance trust among segments of the public in which it has been eroded.

ISSUES FRAMING THE COMMITTEE'S DELIBERATIONS

Information-sharing for databases that have potentially important implications for public health policy and decision-making raises issues that go beyond the traditional norms or practices for analysis and communication of results in science. The objectives of providing public health agencies and the public with guidance for the policy process and of evaluating public health practices place additional responsibilities and demands on those entrusted with protecting the confidentiality of individually identifiable information in the database, agencies acting as gatekeepers, and individuals seeking access to the information. Procedures for access, analysis, and data sharing must foster public trust and confidence in conclusions and decisions based on findings. They should also promote confidence in the integrity and appropriateness of the data for addressing policy-relevant questions. Those goals are more likely to be achieved for vaccine safety issues and the use of the VSD if the procedures are transparent, fair, credible, reliable, and justifiable (Ball et al., 1998; Calman, 2002; McComas, 2004b; McComas and Trumbo, 2001). Concomitantly, the integrity of the data must be monitored and ensured in ways that promote further sharing for the purposes of improving public health by private entities that have access to otherwise unavailable data and resources. Those principles and balancing factors framed the committee's deliberations, its review of current practices, and its recommendations.

Concerns about access to VSD data and the results based on those data are tied closely to concerns about credibility, transparency, and trust regarding the NIP. Trust in the VSD—as a program designed, implemented, and maintained in the public interest—suffers when members of the public do not have confidence that systems for access are fair and transparent. Confidence in the NIP and its public health decisions that touch the lives of millions of Americans is tied directly to the perceived independence, transparency, and fairness of the VSD data sharing program.

PREVIOUS RELEASE OF PRELIMINARY FINDINGS FROM THE VACCINE SAFETY DATALINK

To appreciate the context of the committee's review of whether, when, and how preliminary findings from the VSD should be shared with other scientists, communicated to the public, and used to make policy or recommendations to CDC, it is important to understand the concerns and circumstances surrounding previous releases of preliminary findings from the VSD. Many of the concerns related to the release of preliminary findings from the VSD stem from a study by Verstraeten et al. (2003a) that was intended as an initial screen of possible associations between thimerosal and neurodevelopmental disorders.

Some members of the general public have criticized the thimerosal screening study for changes in the original study protocol, changes in eligibility criteria, the selective official release of preliminary findings, and the inclusion of vaccine manufacturers' representatives in a meeting intended to provide external expert review of the study (Bernard, 2004). One of the publicly expressed criticisms was that preliminary findings indicating no association between thimerosal exposure and neurodevelopmental disorders were released to advocates and at a conference presentation in May 2000, whereas preliminary findings that indicated a weak association were released a month later at the Simpsonwood meeting that included vaccine "insiders" (Bernard, 2004). Concerns about those differences in interpretation have been cited as the reason that a FOIA request was submitted to gain additional information about the study (SafeMinds,

STUDY BACKGROUND AND CONTEXTUAL ISSUES

2003). In a presentation to the committee, NIP staff described the decisions that were made during the course of the thimerosal study, the preliminary findings that were released to particular groups, and the timing of the releases (DeStefano, 2004).

The committee was not charged with reviewing the procedures used for that study, but it was asked to examine the preliminary findings issue by using it and other studies as illustrative examples of the iterative analysis approaches used for VSD studies. The concerns expressed by some members of the general public about such iterative analyses provide a part of the context for the committee's recommendations. A detailed chronology of milestones of two VSD studies is provided later in this report (see Chapter 4).

HOW TRUST AFFECTS THE VACCINE SAFETY DATALINK

Importance of Trust in Perceptions of Vaccine Safety

Trust is essential to risk perceptions of the public and effective risk communication. Trust is easy to lose and difficult to win back (Poortinga and Pidgeon, 2004; Siegrist and Cvetkovich, 2001; Slovic, 1993), and a lack of trust can change how safety information is evaluated. "Negative" events (such as media reports that raise questions about vaccine safety) generally are likely to be weighed more than "positive" information (Cvetkovich et al., 2002; Siegrist and Cvetkovich, 2001). That implies that a single event questioning vaccine safety, even if invalid, can harm parents' confidence in the safety of vaccines (Poortinga and Pidgeon, 2004). People reevaluate their risk perceptions under some circumstances, and confidence can erode even if data suggesting a risk are not overwhelming and are later refuted (Offit and Coffin, 2003).

Generally, Americans have confidence in CDC's and FDA's ability to provide safe and effective vaccines. A recent national survey found that the vast majority of parents (87%) understand the benefits of immunizations and rate immunization safety as relatively high (Gellin et al., 2000). However, a substantial proportion of parents (25%) do have beliefs that could erode their confidence in immunizations (Gellin et al., 2000). One of those beliefs is that children receive more vaccinations than are good for them. Furthermore, recent data from the National Immunization Survey showed that although most parents understand the importance of immunizations, the majority of parents do have some concerns about vaccine safety and have raised this issue with pediatricians (Bardenheier et al., 2004). Those concerns were not enough for most parents to refuse immunizations, but for some groups that was the case. Some American children remain underimmunized (Bardenheier et al., 2004; Gust et al., 2004). In

England, mass-media reports of a study that found a possible link between autism and measles-mumps-rubella vaccine led to decreased immunization rates in England (Offit and Coffin, 2003).

Even though rates of immunization among U.S. children are high, this does not necessarily mean that concerns about vaccine safety are limited to a small percentage of parents that hesitate to immunize their children. A silent majority generally have high confidence in CDC and in immunizations (e.g., Gellin et al., 2000) but also share some of the serious concerns of the more vocal and active groups questioning the safety of vaccines in the United States (Bardenheier et al., 2004; Gellin et al., 2000). Their lingering concerns suggest that building the public's confidence and addressing attitudes and beliefs that might place immunization decisions at risk are crucial tasks for maintaining and improving immunization coverage in the United States (Gust et al., 2004).

Trust Relationships Relevant to the VSD

The committee heard that some people do not trust the NIP to portray vaccine safety risks accurately (Bernard, 2004; Fisher, 2004a). Taking steps to improve the independence, transparency, and fairness of VSD procedures while continuing to protect confidentiality will help to enhance a variety of trust relationships.

Four types of trust relationships are particularly relevant to the VSD, each with specific concerns and implications:

- Researcher-participant
- Researcher-other scientist
- Researcher-society
- Researcher-sponsor

Researcher-participant trust relationships are affected by participants' trust that their personal information will remain confidential (Weijer, 2004). For the VSD, if members of the MCOs that participate in the VSD do not trust that their medical information will remain confidential when analyzed by external (or internal) researchers, MCOs may question their involvement with the VSD since it affects their relationships with their members.

Researcher-other scientist trust relationships are affected by researchers' trust in colleagues to report research results accurately and appropriately (Weijer, 2004). For the VSD, when researchers do not trust that other researchers conducted a study appropriately or reported the results accurately, they may ask to conduct an audit or reanalysis of a published study through the data sharing program.

STUDY BACKGROUND AND CONTEXTUAL ISSUES 23

Researcher-society trust relationships are affected by society's trust in the researchers to portray research findings accurately and to be free of conflicts of interest relevant to the research (Weijer, 2004). For the VSD, if members of the public do not trust that final research results portray all study findings accurately, they may ask to see earlier versions of the study's findings or to have broader access to VSD data.

Researcher-sponsor relationships also must be recognized. The relationship between the sponsor of research and the researcher is relevant to understanding any possible influence on the research—the framing of the research question, the methods used, the interpretation of the findings, and the dissemination of the findings.

Research with VSD data—and scientific research in general—operates best in an environment of trust among all those responsible for and affected by the research findings. The importance of these trust relationships is conveyed in *On Being a Research Scientist* (NAS, NAE, and IOM, 1996):

> The scientific research enterprise, like other human activities, is built on a foundation of trust. Scientists trust that the results reported by others are valid. Society trusts that the results of research reflect an honest attempt by scientists to describe the world accurately and without bias. The level of trust that has characterized science and its relationship with society has contributed to a period of unparalleled scientific productivity. But this trust will endure only if the scientific community devotes itself to exemplifying and transmitting the values associated with ethical scientific conduct.

Trust in sources, trust in researchers, trust in policy, and trust in outcomes all are relevant to the VSD. All are interrelated and affect each other. All can be enhanced by greater trust in the VSD process—the first step in enhancing trust in the findings from the VSD and other vaccine safety activities.

OVERARCHING PRINCIPLES

In the course of its deliberations, the committee found that four overarching principles emerged. The principles can be described as common themes inherent in the committee's recommendations and thus principles that should be considered in any modifications to the VSD data sharing program or any determinations about whether, when, and how to release VSD preliminary findings. The overarching principles apply to issues related both to the VSD data sharing program (the focus of the first part of the committee's charge) and to whether, when, and how to release preliminary findings (the focus of the second part of the charge). The committee's recommendations can be understood best in the context of the four overarching principles.

Some principles are inherent in the scientific process (such as scientific integrity, protection of human subjects, and ethical conduct of research); such principles also are inherent to the VSD research process. The four overarching principles identified by the committee build on the principles that are inherent in the general scientific process. They represent important concerns for VSD research; their relative importance for other kinds of research will vary.

The four overarching principles that emerged from the committee's recommendations are:

- *Independence.* Ensure that potential biases and potential conflicts of interest are minimized, balanced, or otherwise managed in the design and implementation of all processes, practices, and policies related to the VSD.
- *Transparency.* Ensure that all processes, practices, and policies related to the VSD are developed in the spirit of openness, clearly articulated, and easily available to interested persons or entities, and that any deviations from them are documented and justified.
- *Fairness.* Ensure that all processes, practices, and policies related to the VSD are designed and implemented in a fair manner.
- *Protection of confidentiality.* Ensure that the design and implementation of the VSD protect the confidentiality of individually identifiable information.

The committee determined that it could not adequately address issues of independence, transparency, fairness, and protection of confidentiality without examining how the VSD research process supports or hinders the application of those principles. Concerns that arise about the independence and transparency, in particular, of the general VSD research process spill over into people's perceptions of the independence and transparency of the VSD data sharing program and of the determinations about whether, when, and how to release VSD preliminary findings. The committee believed that it had to consider how the VSD research plan, the setting of priorities among VSD studies, and the VSD peer-review process affect the VSD data sharing program and the release of preliminary findings if it wanted to provide the most appropriate and useful recommendations requested in its charge.

2

Description of the Vaccine Safety Datalink

ROLE OF FDA AND CDC IN ASSESSING VACCINE SAFETY

Vaccine Development and Licensure

The Food and Drug Administration (FDA) is responsible for monitoring the safety of candidate vaccines from preclinical studies through prelicensure clinical trials. When a biologics license application (BLA) is submitted for a specific vaccine, FDA, with advice from the Vaccines and Related Biological Products Advisory Committee (VRBPAC), makes the decision of whether to license the product and its manufacturing establishment. FDA also plays a critical role in the postlicensure surveillance of the safety of the vaccine after approval for its administration to the general public (Ball et al., 2004; Baylor et al., 2004).

When sponsors believe that they have sufficient data to initiate the first Phase 1 clinical trial of the vaccine in humans, they submit an investigational new drug (IND) application to FDA's Center for Biologics Evaluation and Research (CBER). FDA has 30 days to review the IND, which includes information on the rationale for the vaccine, the methods of manufacture, characterization, and the results of relevant preclinical tests of the vaccine's safety, immunogenicity, and (if possible) efficacy in animal models and in vitro models. An important part of the IND is the clinical protocol, which must undergo an ethics review and approval by an Institutional Review Board (IRB). As the vaccine candidate advances stepwise through the clinical-development path of Phase 2 and Phase 3 trials, FDA, through the IND process, monitors its safety profile in conjunction with the IRB(s) that initially approved the trial and (for larger studies) a study-specific data safety monitoring board associated with the trial. If questions or concerns of safety arise during a clinical trial, FDA can put the study on "clinical hold" until the questions are satisfactorily addressed.

In parallel with the clinical-development path, the manufacturers develop processes to move from preparation of pilot vaccine lots to large-scale manufacture of lots that are consistent in characterization and immunogenicity. The large-scale manufacturing process is generally in final form before Phase 3 trials begin. Defined manufacturing methods and well-described tests to control the vaccine at critical steps in the manufacturing process are fundamental to ensure the safety and purity of vaccines and to achieve consistency in manufacture. FDA regulations related to the manufacture, product quality, and clinical testing of vaccines are found in Title 21 of the *Code of Federal Regulations* (CFR).[1] To supplement information contained in the CFR, FDA periodically makes available guidance documents that address various aspects of and issues related to vaccine safety.[2]

If the results of the Phase 1, 2, and 3 clinical trials support the safety, immunogenicity, and efficacy of the vaccine, the manufacturing facility is adequate, and the product of manufacture is consistent, the sponsor can submit a BLA to FDA. After consideration of the data, FDA, with advice from VRBPAC, can license the vaccine. VRBPAC includes public members and non-FDA scientists, clinicians, biostatisticians, and epidemiologists (FDA, 2002).

Postmarket Surveillance of Vaccine Safety

FDA continues to play an important role after licensure by making periodic inspections of the manufacturing facility. It can request results of

---

[1]Some examples of relevant sections of the CFR are: 21 CFR 25, Environmental impact considerations; 21 CFR 50, Protection of human subjects; 21 CFR 56, Institutional Review Boards; 21 CFR 58, Good Laboratory Practice for non-clinical laboratory studies; 21 CFR 201, Labeling; 21 CFR 210, Current Good Manufacturing Practice (GMP) in manufacturing, processing packing or holding of drugs (general); 21 CFR 211, GMP practice for finished pharmaceuticals; 21 CFR 312, Investigational New Drug application; 21 CFR 314.126, Adequate and well-controlled clinical trials; 21 CFR 600, Biological products (general); 21 CFR 601, Licensing; and 21 CFR 610, General biological products standards.

[2]In 21 CFR 600, safety is defined as "the relative freedom from harmful effect to persons affected directly or indirectly, by a product when prudently administered, taking into consideration the characteristics of the product in relation to the condition of the recipient at the time."

the manufacturer's tests for controlling the quality (purity, potency, and safety) of different lots of the vaccine, and it can request that samples be submitted for testing by CBER (FDA, 2002).

One mechanism for continued FDA surveillance of safety is active and passive Phase 4 studies (including studies sometimes agreed to by the sponsor as a condition of FDA licensure). In addition, FDA and the Centers for Disease Control and Prevention (CDC) jointly manage the Vaccine Adverse Events Reporting System (VAERS), a passive pharmacovigilance (that is, vaccinovigilance) system that receives 10,000-15,000 reports of adverse events a year on standardized reporting forms (CDC and FDA, 2003). About 15% of VAERS reports reflect serious adverse events involving life-threatening conditions, hospitalization, permanent disability, or death (CDC and FDA, 2005). VAERS relies on ad hoc reporting from patients (or parents of pediatric patients) and from health care providers. The adverse events reported may or may not be causally associated with the immunization.

VAERS is a valuable tool for detecting signals of potential vaccine adverse reactions, but it cannot be used to make definitive vaccine safety determinations, because reporting is voluntary and thus subject to underreporting and bias. Because the design of VAERS does not allow the definition of a study population (that is, it lacks "denominator data"), adverse event rates cannot be calculated with any precision (CDC and FDA, 2004). VAERS cannot be used for statistically valid analyses of direct links between vaccinations and health outcomes. The U.S. system of medical recordkeeping also does not allow direct links between vaccination and health outcomes, because medical record data are not maintained electronically in a standard format. The Vaccine Safety Datalink (VSD) was created and designed to overcome many of those and other limitations of the data available in 1991.

Other CDC Vaccine Safety Activities

In addition to its joint oversight of VAERS with FDA, CDC plays a critical role in vaccine safety by maintaining the VSD and by performing case-control and other epidemiologic studies in the VSD population and in various other U.S. populations when epidemiologic signals suggest that there may be a problem. CDC has also been a pioneer in helping to develop the (informal) subspecialty of immunization safety by funding seven Clinical Immunization Safety Assessment (CISA) centers throughout the United States. One task of the CISA centers is the standardized assessment of persons who experienced acute vaccine adverse reactions (such as anaphylaxis) to enhance knowledge of the biologic basis of and host risk factors for rare but severe reactions (Pless et al., 2004). CDC also is responsible for monitoring the incidence of vaccine-preventable diseases at the national level (Chen, 2004).

DEVELOPMENT OF THE VACCINE SAFETY DATALINK

In 1991, the Institute of Medicine (IOM) Committee to Review the Adverse Consequences of Pertussis and Rubella Vaccines recognized that there were serious gaps and limitations in the current knowledge of and research capacity for assessing vaccine safety (IOM, 1991). That committee concluded that the infrastructure for vaccine safety surveillance had weaknesses and that research capacity must be improved to facilitate reviews of vaccine safety (IOM, 1991). To address some of those concerns, the National Immunization Program (NIP) promptly moved to support the creation of the VSD, a collaboration with a consortium of several managed care organizations (MCOs) to allow timely investigations of vaccine safety concerns and to allow retrospective vaccine safety studies (Davis, 2004).

The VSD is a unique national resource for evaluating vaccine safety. It began with four MCOs and now includes data on more than 7 million members of eight MCOs (Chen et al., 1997; Davis, 2004), about 3.2% of the U.S. population under 18 years old, and 1.7% of the population 18 years old and older (CDC, 2004d). The data included in the VSD are compiled by computer from the participating MCOs' routine administration of health services; there is no chart review or other verification that the data meet reasonable standards for health research. For example, clinical detail is sparse, and care received outside the MCO is not noted. The VSD database links data on patient characteristics, health outcomes (according to data resulting from inpatient, outpatient, and emergency-room records), and vaccination history (vaccine type, date of vaccination, manufacturer, lot number, and injection site) (Davis, 2004). The VSD can be a valuable tool for the retrospective assessment of vaccine safety because the number of people included is large, they generally receive most of their health services at the MCOs, and demographic, health outcome, and vaccination data are maintained electronically. The VSD includes "denominator" data for the study population (in contrast with the data contained in VAERS), so event rates can be calculated.

The NIP contributes substantial resources to the support of the VSD database, to targeted studies that use VSD data, and to support of the VSD data sharing program. In fiscal year 2004, the NIP supported VSD-related activities with about $13 million and about 8.5 full-time-equivalents personnel within the NIP (CDC, 2004d).

Changes in the VSD Contract Provisions

The VSD was established originally by contracts between CDC and four MCOs. The VSD has been expanded to eight MCOs, which the NIP currently supports through a single comprehensive contract with America's Health Insurance Plans. The contract supports the establishment and maintenance of an infrastructure across the MCOs participating in the VSD that allows scientifically rigorous and efficient monitoring of vaccine safety; creation and compilation of combined electronic files from each of the participating MCOs that link vaccination data, medical outcomes, and other relevant data; and evaluation of selected vaccine safety questions by analysis of the combined data provided by the participating MCOs (CDC, 2004d).

The current VSD contract began in September 2002 and has a performance period of 10 years (CDC, 2004d). The new contract provisions, which introduce several major changes, apply to data from the year 2001 and later. The considerations that prompted the change in contract provisions are unclear. Before September 2002, the automated data files that contained VSD data before 2001 were contract deliverables from the MCOs (CDC, 2004d). Those data files were maintained at CDC and considered a database owned by CDC. With the contract that was renegotiated in 2002, ownership of VSD data generated after December 31, 2000, remains with the MCOs (CDC, 2004d).

COMPLEXITY AND LIMITATIONS OF THE VACCINE SAFETY DATALINK DATABASE

The VSD database is updated annually. The participating MCOs each extract relevant data from multiple administrative databases and merge them to create a generally consolidated picture of the members' vaccination and health histories. The completeness and accuracy of the separate administrative databases—which contain vaccination, outpatient, inpatient, emergency-room, pharmacy, and enrollment-status data at each MCO—vary with the type of data, calendar time, and the MCO. Although VSD investigators have worked to standardize data elements across sites, a working knowledge of the complexities of the VSD database is required to analyze the data properly. Issues of defining people "at risk" for vaccination or health events is especially important in the creation of valid scientific data, and the accuracy of VSD analyses requires careful tracking of the enrollment status of each person on the basis of enrollment files. A strong working knowledge of statistics and epidemiology is critical to ensure correct use of stratification, modeling, adjustment (such as for age), and other means to control the effects of confounders and biases. Furthermore, the size of the database and the multiple factors related to vaccination and confounding health outcomes suggest that skilled statistical programming is needed for this resource to be used appropriately.

The limitations of the administrative datasets for data on vaccinations and health outcomes have led NIP-affiliated and MCO-affiliated VSD investigators to conclude that the VSD database is useful primarily to identify and set priorities among subjects that warrant targeted case-control studies. The case-control studies are intended to provide more reliable data because to conduct the study, charts for individual enrollees are reviewed for completeness, consistency, and accuracy. In the case-control studies, variable definitions and coding conventions are standardized, and problems of missing data or misclassification with respect to exposure and outcomes are substantially reduced through one or more methods of data collection (such as on-site medical-record review, patient interviews or examinations, and surveys). The datasets used in the case-control studies have considerably improved validity and reliability. The data are compiled only with substantial effort at the MCOs and only with access to highly confidential personal information. It is the smaller case-control datasets from published studies that are in principle available to outside researchers for reanalysis studies done after 2000. The chart-reviewed data are not available to external researchers for new studies through the VSD data sharing program. These are datasets that arose specifically from retrospective studies, however, so many assumptions inherent in the study designs cannot be examined without repeating the data collection.

Ability to Do Surveillance with the VSD

The VSD has been described as a tool for timely surveillance of vaccine safety concerns (Davis, 2004). However, the manner in which the VSD data files are constructed restricts its utility for surveillance. The committee finds that the VSD should not be characterized as a resource for active surveillance of vaccine safety matters, because data files from each MCO are added to the VSD only each year (CDC, 2004d), thereby limiting the capacity for active, timely surveillance of vaccine safety matters. The VSD has many advantages over other databases (such as comprehensive data on study and control populations), but support of surveillance, as normally conceived in public health practice and research, is not one of its identifying characteristics. The VSD is a robust database for large retrospective studies so it is a valuable resource for a variety of studies.

Proprietary Concerns About VSD Data

A unique aspect of the VSD compared with other databases supported by CDC is that it is constituted from the administrative databases of several MCOs, privately run organizations operating in a competitive field of health care that may not want their competitors to know the details of their subscriber base or business practices. Most other databases supported by CDC are from CDC-sponsored surveys. One consequence of the use of MCO administrative data is the need for protection of proprietary information. MCOs may want to protect different types of information. The current VSD contract includes provisions to protect proprietary interests in relation to the VSD data sharing program (CDC, 2004e).

The MCOs, the NIP, and the National Center for Health Statistics (NCHS) have acknowledged that MCOs' proprietary concerns affected the design of the VSD data sharing program (Bernier, 2004a; Davis, 2004). The committee was not charged with examining whether proprietary concerns justify some of the limitations but it finds that it is important to recognize the effect of the limitations on the ability of the VSD data sharing program to share data with external researchers.

The MCOs, the NIP, and NCHS sometimes cited the confidentiality of proprietary information in their descriptions of the VSD data sharing program. Throughout this report, when the committee discusses confidentiality, it refers to the confidentiality of individually identifiable information in the VSD; despite its importance, the protection of proprietary information is not implied by the committee's use of *confidentiality* in this report.

THE SHELBY AMENDMENT AND THE INFORMATION QUALITY ACT

Whenever there are questions about public access to and the quality of data collected or supported by the federal government, the applicability of the Shelby Amendment and the Information Quality Act (IQA) must be considered. The Shelby Amendment and the IQA are often viewed as compatible and mutually enforcing in that both promote public access to government information (Copeland and Simpson, 2004), the Shelby Amendment focusing on issues of access and the IQA focusing on issues of quality.

The Shelby Amendment, enacted in October 1998 as part of the Treasury and Postal Section of the Omnibus Consolidated and Emergency Supplemental Appropriations Act for fiscal year 1999 (Pub. L. No. 105-277 [1998]), directed the Office of Management and Budget (OMB) to amend its Circular A-110 to ensure that all data produced under a federal award be made available to the public through the procedures established under the Freedom of Information Act (FOIA) 5 U.S.C. § 552 (GAO, 2004). The revised Circular A-110 says that a FOIA request can be submitted "for research data relating to published research findings produced under an award that were used by the Federal Government in developing an agency action that has the force and effect of law" (OMB, 1999). In that context, research data are defined as "the recorded factual material commonly accepted in the scientific community as necessary to validate research findings, but not any of the following: preliminary analyses, drafts of scientific papers, plans for future research, peer reviews, or communications with colleagues"; findings are considered published if they "are published in a peer-reviewed scientific or technical journal" or if a federal agency "publicly and officially cites the research findings in support of an agency action that has the force and effect of law" (OMB, 1999). The committee recognizes that determining the vaccine safety actions that have the "force and effect of law" (if any) could have implications for access to VSD data if the Shelby Amendment is found to be applicable.

The IQA, enacted in December 2000 as Section 515 of the Treasury and General Government Appropriations Act for fiscal year 2001 (Pub. L. No. 106-554 [2000]), required OMB to issue guidelines that "provide policy and procedural guidance to Federal agencies for ensuring the quality, objectivity, utility, and integrity of information (including statistical information)" disseminated to the public by federal agencies (Information Quality Act 44 U.S.C. § 35904(d)(1) [2001]; Information Quality Act 44 U.S.C. § 3516 [2001]). The IQA also required federal agencies to develop their own information quality guidelines and to establish administrative procedures to allow people to seek correction of information that does not comply with the OMB guidance. The committee recognizes that the IQA could have implications for the ability of members of the public to dispute the quality of VSD studies if the IQA is found to be applicable to such studies.

The committee recognized that the Shelby Amendment and the IQA could have important implications for access to VSD data and preliminary findings from the VSD. The applicability of those laws to the VSD should be explored further. If the Shelby Amendment and the IQA are found to be applicable, they could affect the procedures that are used by external researchers to gain access to VSD data and by members of the public to question the quality of VSD studies.

Recommendation 2.1: The committee recommends that the NIP and NCHS seek legal advice to clarify the applicability of the Shelby Amendment and the Information Quality Act to VSD data and VSD preliminary findings.

3

The Vaccine Safety Datalink Data Sharing Program

DESIGN AND IMPLEMENTATION TO DATE OF THE VACCINE SAFETY DATALINK DATA SHARING PROGRAM

Development of the VSD Data Sharing Program

Until August 2002, Vaccine Safety Datalink (VSD) research was limited to researchers from the National Immunization Program (NIP) and the managed care organizations (MCOs) participating in the VSD. The team of VSD researchers set research priorities, determined which studies to undertake, and planned how studies would be monitored.[1] External researchers could in principle pursue a collaborative research project with any of the VSD researchers at the NIP or the MCOs, but no process had been established to allow use of VSD data outside such a collaborative relationship, and there appear to have been no proposals for broader participation.

Development of the VSD data sharing program began in August 2000, and the program was formally established on August 30, 2002 (CDC, 2004d). The program was developed in an ad hoc way with input from the Department of Health and Human Services, Congress, and the MCOs participating in the VSD because of heightened interest in public access to VSD data (Wharton, 2004). No additional funding was provided to the Centers for Disease Control and Prevention (CDC) to develop such a program. It resembles no other existing data sharing program known to the committee.

---

[1]Personal communication, F. DeStefano, NIP, February 10, 2005.

Proposals Submitted to the VSD Data Sharing Program

As of October 2004, the NIP had received proposals requesting the use of VSD data from a very small number of researchers. In September 2002, the NIP received proposals from one group of researchers for 13 new vaccine safety studies and 11 reanalyses (CDC, 2004d). Those proposals were revised and slightly modified. The first group of researchers visited the National Center for Health Statistics (NCHS) Research Data Center (RDC) in October 2003 and January 2004 (Geier and Geier, 2004) to analyze the VSD data for which their access was approved. In August 2003, the NIP received a proposal from another researcher for a reanalysis of a published VSD study of the association between measles-mumps-rubella and varicella vaccines and type 1 diabetes (CDC, 2004f). The researcher's proposal was complete, but at the time of this writing the researcher had not pursued the next steps in the process.

Challenges in Implementing the VSD Data Sharing Program

CDC experienced several challenges in implementing the VSD data sharing program. At the time of the announcement of the data sharing program, CDC did not have a formal data sharing policy to provide a standard or guide for the VSD program (Wharton, 2004). Congressional interest in the status of the VSD data sharing program brought increased scrutiny and time pressures to the development process. Analytic data files from some previously published VSD studies had not been archived in a standard manner, so it was difficult to respond expeditiously to requests to reanalyze published VSD studies. The scope of the data sharing program also had to satisfy the dual objectives of providing access to VSD data and ensuring the privacy of the personal medical information in the VSD (Wharton, 2004). NIP resources and personnel were challenged by those events and competing demands and by the adversarial environment that soon emerged.

Summary of VSD Data Sharing Program Guidelines

Four successive versions of the VSD data sharing program guidelines for independent external researchers have been released publicly. Each version of the guidelines was intended to provide greater clarification about program requirements and expectations than the version before it. In August 2002, the first version of *Guidelines for Data Sharing Proposals from External Researchers: Vaccine Safety Datalink (VSD) Project* was released (CDC, 2002). The guidelines outlined the process for submitting proposals to the NIP, the suggested proposal elements, and the process for requesting Institutional Review Board (IRB) approval from each of the MCOs whose data would be examined.

In October 2003, CDC released the second version of the guidelines, *Guidelines for Data Sharing Program for External Researchers: Access to CDC's Vaccine Safety Datalink Data* (CDC, 2003a). The second version provided additional details about the process that independent external researchers were to use to request access to VSD data, clarified the difference in access between two categories of VSD data (new vaccine safety studies and re-analyses of published VSD studies), described the provisions governing use of the RDC at NCHS to access VSD data, and laid out requirements for the publication of research based on VSD data.

The third version of the VSD data sharing program guidelines was provided by NCHS after the programmatic responsibility for the data sharing program was transferred from the NIP to NCHS in March 2004 (CDC, 2004d). NCHS decided not to create separate guidelines for access to VSD data but rather used its general *Procedures for Use of the RDC* (CDC, 2004b) document and the accompanying RDC *General Description* document (CDC, 2004c) to serve as the interim guidelines for the VSD data sharing program until those documents could be updated.

On November 18, 2004, NCHS published a *Federal Register* notice and request for comments on *Procedures and Costs for Use of the Research Data Center* (CDC, 2004a). Although this document outlines procedures that apply to all datasets available through the RDC, it also constitutes the fourth version of the VSD data sharing program guidelines because it includes project-specific requirements for VSD data in an appendix to the main document (CDC, 2004a). The *Federal Register* notice includes the information that was contained in the two documents that constituted the third version of the VSD data sharing program guidelines and additional information on the RDC and VSD-specific requirements. NCHS requested public comment on this document. The original deadline for public comment was December 9, 2004 (CDC, 2004a); this deadline was extended to March 1, 2005 (CDC, 2004g). (The *Federal Register* notices can be found in Appendix G.) The new RDC procedures provide additional explanation of the expectations for guest researchers at the RDC and costs for use of the RDC (CDC, 2004a). The new VSD-specific guidelines have additional requirements for information that is to be included in proposals, compared with earlier versions of the guidelines for the VSD data sharing program (CDC, 2004a).

THE VACCINE SAFETY DATALINK DATA SHARING PROGRAM'S ABILITY TO SHARE DATA

The VSD data sharing program does not meet the traditional definition of data sharing, because of the limitations of the data available through the program and the differing levels of access to VSD data that depend on the type of researcher requesting access.

Because of the contract provisions that govern the VSD data sharing program, independent external researchers are unable to gain access to data from the year 2001 or later for new studies (such as investigation of a new hypothesis or use of novel methods to investigate a previously studied hypothesis), whereas researchers affiliated with the NIP or with one of the VSD MCOs have access to these data for all types of studies. Even for new studies conducted by independent external researchers with data from before 2001, the available data are generally less than ideal in that only data from the annual VSD extracts are provided to these researchers; researchers affiliated with the NIP or the MCOs can use chart review or other means to improve the quality of the data used for a particular study.

Data sharing through the VSD data sharing program is also impeded by the requirement, for all reanalyses, to obtain IRB approval from all MCOs whose data are included in the final dataset. If one MCO's IRB does not provide approval, a reanalysis of the full set of study data cannot be done, because the researcher would be analyzing only part of the data used in the original study.

Confidentiality concerns alone may not sufficiently justify those limitations. Any independent external researcher seeking use of VSD data is required to access the data at the NCHS RDC. The RDC is designed to make breaches of confidentiality nearly impossible. The data access restrictions in place at the RDC are sound and extensive, and they reduce the possibility of breaches of confidentiality regardless of the extent or type of data being accessed or the intentions of external researchers.

In preparing its advice to the NIP and NCHS, the committee recognizes the current limitations of the VSD data sharing program. If the NIP and NCHS want to allow access to VSD data in the true spirit of a data sharing program, the committee's advice and recommendations will help the program to meet scientific standards of data sharing. If the current limitations of the program are not overcome, the NIP should characterize the program as a limited data access program rather than a data sharing program. The committee finds that overcoming the limitations may require renegotiation of the VSD contract.

A true VSD data sharing program would need to include the following three elements: access to the core VSD data for exploratory analyses; access to studies that involve chart review, and so on, to consider alternative explanations; and new collaborative studies with the NIP and the MCOs to pursue new hypotheses. If the intention is to allow true data sharing, researchers should be allowed use of all available years of data for new studies and not be limited to final datasets for reanalyses.

The VSD is a public resource that is designed to inform important public health policy decisions. By the very nature of its potential to influence policy, the public demands and deserves access to the data used to influence those decisions and transparency in the processes that permit or restrict access. If the VSD indeed is intended to be used as a foundation of policy decisions, there is a public need to share data fairly and to be as transparent as possible while protecting the confidentiality of individually identifiable information in the VSD.

The committee uses the term *VSD data sharing program* throughout this report for the sake of consistency and ease of reference. Despite the limitations of the sharing function of the VSD data sharing program, the term is now well established.

CURRENT STANDARDS OF PRACTICE OF SIMILAR DATA SHARING PROGRAMS

Benefits and Costs of Sharing Data

Sharing of VSD data or any other type of data has both benefits and costs. Some benefits and costs may be unique to the sharing of particular datasets, but the often-cited benefits of data sharing include (Fienberg, 1994; NRC and the Committee on National Statistics, 1985):

- Reinforcement of open scientific inquiry;
- Verification, refutation, or refinement of original results;
- Promotion of new research through existing data;
- Encouragement of the appropriate use of empirical data in policy formulation and evaluation;
- Improvement of methods for data collection and measurement;
- Development of theoretical knowledge and knowledge of analytic techniques;
- Encouragement of multiple perspectives;
- Provision of resources for training in research;
- Protection against faulty data;
- Greater application of scientific research in decision-making;
- Reduction of the expense of duplicative data collection and the concomitant burden on human subjects; and
- Respect for the desire of respondents to contribute to societal knowledge.

In the case of VSD data, the committee finds that, especially in the context of government-funded research, increased data sharing also promotes greater transparency in the derivation of research results, which enhances public trust in the use of the VSD to make accurate assessments of vaccine safety.

Data sharing also has costs. Those often cited are related to (Fienberg, 1994; NRC and the Committee on National Statistics, 1985):

- Elimination of technical obstacles to sharing data;
- Need for extensive technical and substantive documentation of datasets;
- Monetary and time costs to original researcher for preparing data for sharing;
- Monetary and time costs to subsequent analysts for developing a base of knowledge about the data;
- Response to errors by others;
- Response to unwarranted criticisms based on poor analyses by others;
- Loss of original researchers' exclusive right to future discoveries; and
- Breaches of confidentiality.

The constraints that limit access to VSD data and can be considered costs of the VSD data sharing program include protection of proprietary information, protection of detailed medical information, and protection of intellectual property rights of researchers.

The benefits of, costs of, and risks posed by data sharing are important in examining the VSD data sharing program so that any proposed changes in the program can be understood properly. Expanding or limiting access to VSD data will lead to nontrivial shifts in the balance of costs and benefits. Some of the committee's recommendations promote expanding access to VSD data, and some create constraints on access to VSD data. The NIP and NCHS will have to consider the costs and benefits of the different recommendations to determine which ones to implement.

Approaches to Data Access

Data can be shared in a number of ways—public-use data files (with data elements that are limited or altered to prevent identification of individuals), restricted data use agreements and licensing agreements, and access to restricted data at a data enclave. Many data sources allow access to be granted through multiple means, depending on the sensitivity of the data needed for a particular study.

Public-use data files are available to anyone who would like to use the data. Data providers normally provide a data dictionary and background information on the design features of the data source. Carefully constructed public-use data files present the lowest risk of disclosure of confidential information.

Restricted data use agreements and licensing agreements may allow researchers access to data that are somewhat broader than what is available in public-use data files. To help to ensure that confidential data remain protected, the data owners or data stewards require the researcher to sign a restricted data use or licensing agreement. The agreement specifies the penalties for violating provisions of the agreement.

Access to restricted data at a data enclave allows researchers to use data that are very sensitive or might allow easy identification of individuals whose information is included in the database. To access data at a data enclave, researchers submit a proposal outlining their proposed study and describing why confidential or sensitive data not available in other ways are needed. Researchers conduct their analyses at the data enclave, and all output must be reviewed for the risk of disclosure before it can leave the data enclave.

Review of Similar Data Sharing Programs

To assess how the VSD data sharing program compares with current standards of practice for data sharing in the scientific community, the committee reviewed extensive information about different data sharing policies, different types of data sharing activities, and legal and regulatory provisions governing confidentiality of data. The committee found that the provisions that are in place for data sharing activities reflect increasing concerns about confidentiality and thus increasing restrictions on access to data: public-use data files, restricted data use agreements, and access to confidential data files in a controlled environment (through a data enclave). The committee's recommendations on the specific provisions of the VSD data sharing program reflect its review of current standards of practice for data sharing.

Because the VSD is a unique database, with unique conditions governing its creation and use, no single data sharing program is a perfect model for comparison with it, but the committee identified four data-enclave approaches to data sharing that have operations similar to the VSD data sharing program and have similar concerns, including the need for confidentiality. The committee reviewed those four data sharing programs to assess current standards of practice of programs similar to that of the VSD, although they do not contain the same type of data as the VSD. All those programs allow access to restricted data through a data-enclave approach and have written rules, limitations, application processes, and review processes. Subsets of data, often called public-use data files, are also available from some of those data sources with virtually no restrictions. The data enclaves are for follow-up and access to individually identifiable data in a form that protects confidentiality. Those programs are the Medical Expenditure Panel Survey (MEPS) of the Agency for Healthcare Research and Quality (AHRQ), the program of the Census Bureau RDCs, the Health and Retirement Study (HRS) at the University of Michigan, and the California Health Interview Survey (CHIS). The committee finds that the unique circumstances surrounding the creation, maintenance, and use of the VSD will require that the VSD use some specific adaptations to standard data sharing procedures and practices to account for its unique circumstances.

Description of Data Sharing Provisions for Different Data Enclaves

Table 1 (page 42) summarizes the specific provisions that govern access to restricted data at the data enclaves the committee reviewed in depth.

Medical Expenditure Panel Survey

The MEPS collects detailed data on specific health services used in the United States and allows linkage of different data files (AHRQ, 2004c). Some MEPS data files are available as public-use files, but others can be accessed only in the secure environment of the Center for Financing, Access, and Cost Trends Data Center (CFACT-DC). There is an application process to obtain approval for use of the center and a fee for each use (AHRQ, 2004b). Review of the application includes an evaluation of the feasibility of the researchers' proposal, a review of whether the analysis can be done without breaching confidentiality, a determination of the compatibility of the project with the AHRQ mission, and the availability of resources within the CFACT-DC for whatever work may be needed to respond to the request (AHRQ, 2004b). Staff resources to provide assistance at the CFACT-DC are limited, so extensive programming support must be contracted ahead of time for a fee. The manager at the CFACT-DC coordinates the review of each proposal. Once a proposal is approved, the researchers can access the data by going to the CFACT-DC at AHRQ to access the files (AHRQ, 2004a). That usually occurs about 4-6 weeks after approval. Researchers can access only the variables that were identified and approved in their proposal (AHRQ, 2004d). All materials must be reviewed by AHRQ staff before they can be removed from the data center.

Census Bureau Research Data Centers

The Census Bureau RDCs allow researchers to carry out research with confidential census records. The external research program is supported by the Center for Economic Studies (CES), and its data records are available to "sophisticated" users in a controlled and secure environment (Census Bureau, 2004b). Researchers must register as potential users with CES through the Census Bureau Web site, and their proposal can then be submitted through the same Web site (Census Bureau, 2004a). Each proposal must identify a specific dataset to be analyzed and show that the research can be conducted successfully with the proposed methods and the data available. The proposal must show the need for and importance of using confidential data, and researchers who will have access to confidential data must obtain "special sworn status" from the Census Bureau. In this case, special sworn status requires passing a security clearance and signing a statement agreeing to preserve the confidentiality of the data (Census Bureau, 2004a). Researchers can use confidential data only for the purpose for which the data are supplied or pursuant to the objectives of Title 13, which authorizes the Census Bureau to collect such data, and all analyses must be done at the RDC. All proposals need to gain approval from both the RDC and the Census Bureau and must demonstrate a benefit to the bureau's programs (Census Bureau, 2004b). The RDC administrator reviews preliminary proposals and may suggest ways to improve and refine them. The administrator must approve a preliminary proposal before researchers can submit the final proposal. Researchers should expect a minimum of a 6-month lapse between submitting their final proposal and the commencement of research with confidential data (Census Bureau, 2004a). All data to be taken out of the RDC must go through a disclosure review; no confidential data can be taken out of the center. Researchers must undergo a security check before leaving the RDC (Census Bureau, 2004b).

Health and Retirement Study

The HRS at the University of Michigan includes information that is made available to external researchers only under strict conditions (HRS, 2004a). The datasets from the HRS are cleaned and processed to make use easier and are supplemented with information files provided by users (HRS, 2004a). The HRS Web site lists what data will be made available for study and analysis (HRS, 2004c). To use HRS data, researchers must submit a research proposal package. The researchers must identify a dataset of interest and state why the unrestricted data will not be adequate for the research purpose. They must also submit a restricted data protection plan to the HRS. Reviewers consider the risk of disclosure of restricted information on the basis of the users' description of expected analysis, the scientific and technical feasibility of the project, the availability of data files being requested, and whether the proposed project is in accordance with

TABLE 1 Comparison of Data Sharing Programs That Use Data Enclaves

	Medical Expenditure Panel Survey (MEPS)	Census Research Data Centers (RDCs)
GENERAL INFORMATION ON THE DATA SHARING PROGRAMS		
Type of Data	MEPS is the third (and most recent) in a series of national probability surveys conducted by AHRQ on the financing and use of medical care in the United States. MEPS collects data on the specific health services that Americans use, how frequently they use them, the costs of the services, how they are paid, and the cost, scope, and breadth of private health insurance held by and available to the U.S. population.	Census data include microdata and data that cannot be released publicly, because they contain detailed information on geographic location and other characteristics about the firms or households that could be used to determine their identities.
ELEMENTS OF STUDY PROPOSAL		
Identification of Specific Variables to Be Studied	▶ Researchers must list data files to which they would like access to. ▶ Researchers will have access only to the variables identified in their approved proposals.	▶ Researchers must identify the specific dataset to be analyzed.

Health and Retirement Study (HRS)	California Health Interview Survey (CHIS)	Vaccine Safety Datalink (VSD) *based on 2004 *Federal Register* Notice*
The University of Michigan HRS surveys more than 22,000 Americans over the age of 50 every 2 years. The survey collects data on respondents' physical and mental health, insurance coverage, financial status, family support systems, labor-market status, and retirement planning. Registered users can download HRS public data products free. Restricted-release files contain sensitive information that can be made available only under specified conditions.	CHIS is a telephone survey of adults, adolescents, and children from all parts of the state of California. The survey is conducted every 2 years. Some of the data collected are prepared for public release as free public-use files. The files are designed to minimize the risk of respondent identification yet preserve the broadest range of descriptive demographic data. Restricted-use files at CHIS available at the DAC contain detailed geographic identifiers and full demographic descriptions for the survey respondents from the 2001 survey. The files also include responses to sensitive questions that are excluded from the public-use data files.	The VSD is a large linked database that was developed in 1991 by the collaborative efforts of CDC and several private MCOs. The VSD currently includes data from administrative records for more than 7 million members of eight MCOs. In the VSD, vaccination records, patient characteristics, and health outcomes are linked, allowing the VSD to serve as a unique and potentially powerful resource for the continuing evaluation of vaccine safety.
▶ A specific dataset must be chosen from the list of restricted-use datasets. ▶ Researchers must state why the unrestricted data would not be adequate for their research purpose.	▶ Researchers must request variables using the DAC variable lists.	▶ Researchers must provide a list detailing data requested: data system, files, years, and variables. ▶ Only variables needed to conduct the proposed analyses will be included in the analytic file.

Continued

TABLE 1 Continued

	Medical Expenditure Panel Survey (MEPS)	Census Research Data Centers (RDCs)
Confidentiality Protection Measures in Study Design	▶ The proposed study must be done without compromising confidentiality of respondents. ▶ Researchers must read and comply with the CFACT-DC User Guide.	▶ Researchers must obtain Special Sworn Status. ▶ Researchers can use confidential data only for the purpose for which the data are supplied.
Feasibility of Study and Data-Resource Assessment	Decision Criteria: ▶ Can the research be conducted with the available data?	▶ The proposal must show that the research can be conducted successfully with the proposed method and available data. ▶ The proposal should show the need for and importance of using confidential data.

Health and Retirement Study (HRS)	California Health Interview Survey (CHIS)	Vaccine Safety Datalink (VSD) *based on 2004 *Federal Register* Notice*
▶ Researchers must submit a Restricted Data Protection Plan to HRS. ▶ Risk of disclosure of restricted information is considered based on the users' description of expected analysis and results. ▶ The Confidentiality Agreement Restricting Disclosure and Use of Data from the Michigan Center on the Demography of Aging Data Enclave must be read and signed by the researchers. ▶ All users will be periodically audited by HRS to ensure that all conditions of the Restricted Data Agreement are being met. Various data from 1992-2004 are available.	Decision Criteria: ▶ Is there a risk of disclosure of confidential information? ▶ Does the project propose to merge user-supplied data with CHIS data? ▶ What additional risks of disclosure are associated with the merged dataset? ▶ Researchers must sign a Nondisclosure Affidavit and Data Access Confidentiality Agreement before starting their work.	▶ All users must sign an affidavit of confidentiality promising not to attempt to identify respondents. ▶ All users must sign an agreement regarding the conditions of access to confidential data in the RDC. ▶ Researchers can use confidential data only for the purpose for which the data are supplied.
▶ Scientific and technical feasibility of the project, including availability of data files being requested, is considered.	Decision Criteria: ▶ Is sample size sufficient? ▶ Are CHIS data appropriate for answering the research questions proposed? ▶ Are the variables requested related to the proposed analyses?	▶ No criteria specified for review of VSD proposals. ▶ No publicly available data.

Continued

TABLE 1 Continued

	Medical Expenditure Panel Survey (MEPS)	Census Research Data Centers (RDCs)
Consistency with Mission of the Organization	▶ The proposed study must be in accordance with the mission of AHRQ (this is specified in its authorizing legislation).	▶ All projects must provide a benefit to Census Bureau programs. The benefit requirement is an explicit proposal criterion and is required by law (Title 13, Sec. 23, U.S.C.).
IRB Approval	(Information not available.)	▶ The need for IRB approval is based on the source of the confidential data, and the researchers must follow the rules and regulations of that agency.

OTHER GUIDELINES

Costs and Fees	▶ At the data center: To cover technical assistance, simple file construction, and up to 2 hours of programming support, there is a $150.00 fee. Additional programming support can cost $80.00 an hour.	▶ $3,125/month for full-time use. ▶ A project that requires a 40% level of access (about 2 days/week) for a period of 1 year would cost $15,000. ▶ Additional fees may be charged to projects that use datasets outside the core or that impose other special costs on CES, the Census Bureau, or the RDC.

Health and Retirement Study (HRS)	California Health Interview Survey (CHIS)	Vaccine Safety Datalink (VSD) *based on 2004 *Federal Register* Notice*
▶ Proposed project must be in accordance with the mission of the MiCDA.	▶ Study must be compatible with the purpose of CHIS.	▶ Not specified for VSD data.
▶ Researchers must be affiliated with an institution with an NIH-certified Human Subjects Review Process. ▶ A signed form from the researchers' institution certifying Human Subjects Review was done is necessary.	▶ Copy of approval or exemption by home institution's IRB is necessary.	▶ Researchers must obtain IRB approval from each MCO whose data they would need to undertake the analyses.
▶ Academic (faculty members of accredited institutions of higher education) or government (federal, state, or local): $200/day. ▶ Student (currently enrolled in an accredited graduate or undergraduate program): $50/day. ▶ Other: $500/day.	Costs are developed on an individual basis and include: ▶ $500 initial set-up fee. ▶ $65/hour for guest research access. ▶ $140/hour for programming services. ▶ $120/hour to run programs. ▶ $1,000 minimum fee per project. Charges are determined by actual time spent on project.	▶ Setup charge of $500/day for merging files or creating custom file formats. ▶ Guest researchers: $200/day (2-day minimum, 10-day maximum).

Continued

TABLE 1 Continued

	Medical Expenditure Panel Survey (MEPS)	Census Research Data Centers (RDCs)
Who Reviews Researchers' Application and Proposal?	▶ The manager at the CFACT-DC coordinates the review of each proposal.	▶ Both the RDC and the Census Bureau must approve the proposal. ▶ The RDC administrator reviews the preliminary proposal and suggests ways to improve or refine it. The RDC administrator must approve the preliminary proposal before the researchers can submit the final proposal.
Response Time	▶ Applications are accepted continuously. ▶ About 4-6 weeks after proposal is approved, researchers can go into the CFACT-DC.	▶ There is at least a 6-month period between the deadline for the final proposal submission and the commencement of research.

Health and Retirement Study (HRS)	California Health Interview Survey (CHIS)	Vaccine Safety Datalink (VSD) *based on 2004 *Federal Register* Notice*
▶ The HRS DCC-WG reviews the application. When the application is adequate, the DCC-WG will contact the researchers and let them know that they can submit the application to their local IRB for review. Once the researchers have IRB approval, their application is complete, and they can submit it for review by the DCC for review and final approval.	▶ DAC staff prepares a summary of the application. The CHIS Data Disclosure Review Committee meets biweekly, reviews the application, and makes a recommendation to the CHIS Principle Investigator to approve or reject the application or to request further information from the researchers.	▶ For NCHS data, completed proposals are sent to the NCHS RDC for review by a committee consisting of the director of NCHS RDC, the RDC staff liaison, the NCHS Confidentiality Officer, and the director of the NCHS data division whose data are included in the proposal. ▶ Process not specified for VSD data. ▶ Approval for use of the VSD requires approval by the MCOs' IRBs.
▶ When HRS receives an application, it is logged and review is scheduled.	▶ The CHIS Principle Investigator will respond to the request within 21 days after receiving the application. ▶ Computer programs that are e-mailed to the DAC staff will be run within 5 working days.	▶ Response time varies but NCHS tries to respond to the initial proposal as soon as possible. ▶ The time it takes between securing proposal approval and using the RDC varies as well (depends on the complexity of the work, how long it will take to prepare the data files, and what other work is already scheduled at the RDC).

Continued

TABLE 1 Continued

	Medical Expenditure Panel Survey (MEPS)	Census Research Data Centers (RDCs)
Assistance from Program Staff	▶ Currently, there are limited staff resources to help at the CFACT-DC, so extensive programming support must be contracted ahead of time for a fee.	▶ Researchers work closely with the RDC administrator to develop a preliminary proposal.
Available Data Programs	SAS, Stata, SPSS, and SUDAAN are the software packages most suitable for analyzing MEPS data.	(Information not available.)

Health and Retirement Study (HRS)	California Health Interview Survey (CHIS)	Vaccine Safety Datalink (VSD) *based on 2004 *Federal Register* Notice*
▶ MicDA-DC users are responsible for developing and implementing all data-management procedures necessary to produce datasets to be used for analysis. ▶ MicDA-DC staff provide assistance with dataset installation, software installation, operating-system problems, statistical-package operation, backups, and user-interface issues. ▶ Staff members do not provide assistance in carrying out statistical analysis.	▶ Researchers are encouraged to consult the DAC manager while developing their proposals. ▶ Researchers are provided with limited technical assistance on CHIS variables, weighting, and variance calculation. ▶ A senior programmer contact is assigned to the project. ▶ Dummy data files are sent to the researchers.	▶ Researchers are encouraged to check with RDC staff before writing their proposals to ensure that the data of interest can be made available to them. ▶ Researchers must be able to conduct their analyses with the software specified in their research proposal.
Stata (v6.0), SAS (v6.12), SPSS (v9.0).	SAS, SPSS, Stata, STAT/Transfer, SUDAAN, and Wesvar; custom software is installed on request.	Hardware: Pentium computers with Windows 2000. SAS is the standard program for use of VSD data, but other languages can be made available with sufficient lead time.

Continued

TABLE 1 Continued

	Medical Expenditure Panel Survey (MEPS)	**Census Research Data Centers (RDCs)**
Where Data Can Be Accessed	▶ Public-use datasets can be downloaded from the MEPS Web site (http://www.meps.ahrq.gov). ▶ Restricted data can be accessed by approved researchers at the CFACT-DC, in Rockville, MD. ▶ Researchers may also choose to contract with the AHRQ data-processing contractor (Social and Scientific Systems) to develop and run their programs.	▶ All analysis must be done on site in the RDC.
Disclosure Review Before Material Leaves the RDC	▶ All materials must be reviewed by AHRQ staff before they can be removed from the data center.	▶ Researchers cannot remove any confidential data from the RDC on any medium. All output must be submitted to Census Bureau personnel for disclosure review.

Health and Retirement Study (HRS)	California Health Interview Survey (CHIS)	Vaccine Safety Datalink (VSD) *based on 2004 *Federal Register* Notice*
▶ Public-use files can be accessed through the HRS Web site (http://hrsonline.isr.umich.edu/data/avail.html). ▶ Restricted-use data can be viewed by approved researchers at MiCDA data enclave in the Institute for Social Research.	▶ Public-use files can be accessed through the CHIS Web site by registering for free (http://www.chis.ucla.edu/main/default.asp?page=puf). ▶ Restricted data can be viewed at the DAC at the UCLA Center for Health Policy Research after submitting and gaining approval of a proposal. ▶ Researchers can also gain access to restricted files after proposal approval by e-mailing computer programs to DAC staff, who will run them and send results to the researchers.	▶ All analyses must be done on site in the RDC in Hyattsville, MD. ▶ A maximum of three collaborating researchers can sit at a computer station at the RDC.
▶ Users are allowed to remove results of statistical analysis from the data enclave only after enclave staff have conducted a disclosure-limitation review to protect respondent confidentiality.	▶ DAC manager or senior programmer conducts a disclosure review for all output before it is removed from the DAC.	▶ All output and materials removed from the RDC are subject to disclosure-limitation review. ▶ Researchers must provide a list of the table shells, needed equations, and test statistics of statistical output they plan to take out of the RDC.

Continued

TABLE 1 Continued

	Medical Expenditure Panel Survey (MEPS)	Census Research Data Centers (RDCs)
Other Requirements	Researchers must also provide: ▶ List of publication plans and other intended uses of data in the proposal. ▶ Sources of funding. ▶ Estimated timeframe for viewing data and completing their work. ▶ Resumes or CVs for all persons who will access the data center.	Researchers must also provide: ▶ Purpose of the research. ▶ Funding source. ▶ CVs for all investigators. ▶ Abstract of the proposal. ▶ Project description. ▶ Statement of benefits to Census Bureau. Preliminary and final proposals are completed through the Census Bureau Web site.
Postapplication Activities	(Information not available.)	▶ Once a proposal is approved, all researchers must go through a background investigation. ▶ Researchers are asked (but not required) to work with the RDC administrator before releasing final output.

SOURCES: AHRQ, 2004a,b,c,d; CDC, 2004a; Census Bureau, 2004a,b; CHIS, 2003; CHIS, 2004a,b; HRS, 2004a,b,c; Personal Communication, K. Harris and J. Madans, NCHS, February 9, 2005.

THE VACCINE SAFETY DATALINK DATA SHARING PROGRAM

Health and Retirement Study (HRS)	California Health Interview Survey (CHIS)	Vaccine Safety Datalink (VSD) *based on 2004 *Federal Register* Notice*
▶ If institutional or physical circumstances of the researchers change, HRS is to be contacted to modify the underlying agreement. ▶ Yearly recertification of the certification and data agreement is required. ▶ Researchers must submit a renewal request if initial agreement expires and they want continued access to the data. Researchers must also provide: ▶ Current resume, or CVs. ▶ Dates of proposed tenure at the data enclave. ▶ Funding sources for user project and for data enclave cost recovery. (Information not available.)	If there are many small cells, the programmer recommends the recoding of variables so that this does not occur. If there are few small cells in the output, the programmer must suppress small cells and do complementary suppression. DAC applications include: ▶ DAC application forms. ▶ Personal and organizational information. ▶ Service request. ▶ Abstract. Supplemental Materials include: ▶ Biographic sketch or resume. ▶ List of CHIS variables requested. ▶ Detailed description of any user-supplied files. Researchers must also: ▶ Acknowledge CHIS in their manuscript for publication. ▶ Submit copies of publications to DAC.	Researchers must also provide: ▶ Current Resume or CVs. ▶ Dates of proposed use of the RDC. ▶ Source of funding. ▶ Summary of proposed study. ▶ Background of the study. ▶ Data dictionary. NCHS complies with 308(d) Confidentiality Statute. ▶ External researchers are required to submit a copy of the data-sharing guidelines and a copy of the signed confidentiality agreement with any manuscript submitted to a journal. ▶ Must include certain disclaimers in their manuscript.

the mission of the Michigan Center on the Demography of Aging (MiCDA).

Each application is logged, and a schedule for review is developed. The HRS Data Confidentiality Committee Working Group (DCC-WG) reviews the application first. When that group has approved the application, it informs the researchers that the proposal is ready for review by the local IRB. Once the researchers have IRB approval, the application is considered complete, and they can submit it for review by the DCC-WG for review and final approval (HRS, 2004b). Researchers with approved proposals can view the data at the MiCDA data enclave in the Institute for Social Research. Enclave users are responsible for developing and implementing all data-management procedures necessary to produce the datasets to be used for analysis. Enclave staff provide assistance with dataset installation, software installation, operating-system problems, statistical-package operation, backups, and user-interface issues. Staff members do not assist in statistical analysis. Users are allowed to remove results of statistical analysis from the data enclave only after enclave staff have conducted a disclosure limitation review to protect respondent confidentiality.

California Health Interview Survey

The CHIS is a telephone survey conducted in all areas of California that collects extensive information on health status, health conditions, health-related behaviors, health insurance coverage, and other matters (CHIS, 2004a). Adults, adolescents, and children are included. The data include detailed geographic identifiers and full demographic descriptions of survey respondents (CHIS, 2004b). To view CHIS data, researchers must request specific variables from the Data Access Center (DAC) variable lists. Approval for use of the data is based on feasibility of the proposal (for example, adequacy of sample size, whether CHIS data are appropriate to answer the proposed question, and whether requested variables are related to the proposed analyses), risk of disclosure of confidential information, and compatibility of the proposal with the purpose of the CHIS (Habte, 2004). In addition, researchers must sign a nondisclosure affidavit and data access confidentiality agreement before starting work. Researchers are encouraged to consult the DAC manager as they develop their proposals, and a senior programmer contact is assigned to the project. Researchers are provided with limited technical assistance on CHIS variables, weighting, and variance calculation. Dummy data files are sent to researchers for practice in using the data. The CHIS Data Disclosure Review Committee, which meets every 2 weeks, reviews applications and makes recommendations to approve or reject the application or to request further information from the researchers (Habte, 2004). The principal investigator generally will respond to the request within 21 days after receiving the application. The data can be accessed at the DAC at the University of California, Los Angeles Center for Health Policy Research, which, like the other data centers described earlier, is a secure and controlled environment (Habte, 2004). Researchers can access only data for which their proposals were approved. All materials are inspected before they can be taken out of the CHIS data center.

Current Standards of Practice for Data Enclaves

Independent external researchers are allowed access to VSD data only through the RDC at NCHS. The RDC is a statistical data enclave where data may be more freely accessed (although still under rigorous controls) provided that only approved statistical summaries leave the enclave.

The VSD is a unique and complex database that requires special circumstances for use, but lessons can be learned from the data sharing programs described above. The four programs reviewed by the committee have many common characteristics that the committee finds to be relevant to the VSD data sharing program:

- Researchers must be specific about the variables needed.
- Researchers must justify the need for and relevance of confidential data and state why public data will not suffice.
- Researchers must provide a plan to protect the confidentiality of the individually identifiable information in the dataset.
- Final proposals must be reviewed for feasibility, relevance to the purpose or mission of the organization, and risk of disclosure of confidential information.
- A responsible person or board oversees a defined proposal review process.
- IRB approval is required.
- Researchers access data at designated data enclaves.
- Only minimal data analysis assistance, if any, is offered; limited technical assistance is available in the data center.
- Disclosure review for all information taken out of the data enclave is required.

The committee used the common characteristics to compare the VSD data sharing program with current standards of practice and to guide its findings, conclusions, and recommendations.

Alternative Data Sharing Models to Consider

The RDC uses a variety of procedures to ensure that the confidentiality of data is protected. The committee has reviewed the general policies of the NCHS RDC and finds them to be reasonably reflective of generally recognized professional statistical standards, given the confidentiality concerns of the data because of the different types of linkable data that are available on individuals in the VSD database.

Even though the NIP, NCHS, and the MCOs have decided to use the data enclave model of the NCHS RDC to allow access to VSD data, other data sharing models could be considered. Offering data through a restricted data use agreement or licensing model could be feasible as an alternative model for sharing VSD data. The committee finds that this alternative model could protect confidentiality of individually identifiable data although the mechanism for ensuring confidentiality in this model (the threat of prosecution for breaches of confidentiality) is less stringent than the mechanism used in the data-enclave model (disclosure review to ensure that no identifiable data leave the data enclave). A restricted data use agreement model would reduce the burden on interested external researchers, although it potentially creates a greater risk of disclosure of confidential information. The committee believes that an evaluation of the appropriateness and user-friendliness of alternative data sharing models for the VSD is reasonable and that alternative data sharing models should not be rejected without further consideration of their benefits, risks, and costs.

FRAMEWORK OF RECOMMENDATIONS ON ACCESS TO VACCINE SAFETY DATALINK DATA

Reflecting on all the information gathered throughout its study, the committee finds that the VSD data sharing program has three short-term goals:

1. To facilitate access to and use of the VSD;
2. To protect the confidentiality of individually identifiable data in the VSD; and
3. To enhance public trust in the VSD as a tool to address specific concerns about vaccine safety.

On the basis of those three goals, the committee developed its recommendations in the following framework:

- The NIP should support the broadest feasible use of the VSD for

vaccine safety research within the constraints of law, protection of confidentiality, and VSD contract provisions;
- Bureaucratic and technical barriers to accessing the VSD should be minimized, although some types of studies may require collaboration with or facilitation by data custodians;
- Guidelines for proposals from independent external researchers should be developed and publicized to facilitate access;
- Responses to proposals should be timely;
- Criteria for the independent review of proposals should be publicly accessible;
- Costs to researchers should approximate the incremental costs of access;
- Descriptions of the objectives and methods of current and published studies should be made publicly available;
- All VSD users should provide a timely and detailed public report of their results to the NIP; and
- All completed VSD studies should be subjected to scientific peer review before any public release.

LIMITATIONS OF DATA AVAILABLE THROUGH THE VACCINE SAFETY DATALINK DATA SHARING PROGRAM

The VSD data sharing program allows external researchers to submit a proposal to conduct new vaccine safety studies with the pre-2001 VSD data files that reside at CDC or reanalyze study-specific final datasets from some VSD published studies (CDC, 2004a).

Limitations of the Data Available to External Researchers for New Studies

The November 2004 version of the guidelines states that external researchers can conduct new vaccine safety studies "from the VSD data files that reside at CDC" (CDC, 2004a). Later in the guidelines, it is explained that "VSD data files contain data through December 31, 2000" (CDC, 2004a). Data that were included in the VSD only before the contract renegotiation in 2002 (data for events through the year 2000) are considered "VSD data files that reside at CDC." Therefore, only VSD data for events before January 1, 2001, are available for new vaccine safety studies through the VSD data sharing program. The committee finds that that important provision limiting the data available to independent external researchers for new vaccine studies is not sufficiently clear and explicit in the current version of the VSD data sharing guidelines.

Recommendation 3.1: The committee recommends that future revisions of the VSD data sharing guidelines clearly and explicitly describe the VSD data that are and are not available to independent external researchers for new vaccine studies through the VSD data sharing program.

Quality of Data Available for New Studies

A hypothesis of interest to VSD investigators affiliated with the NIP or one of the participating MCOs might first be examined by using the automated data at one or more of the participating MCOs. Such studies (that use the automated data) estimate associations between particular vaccine exposures and the outcomes of interest. Once the appropriate design considerations have been determined (such as case definitions and exposure categories), the studies can be readily conducted with the existing databases. However, they are limited by all the shortcomings of the underlying administrative databases, including possibly incomplete or potentially biased capture of exposure or outcome information and minimal information on potential confounders. The effects of such problems vary with study population, exposure, outcome, and calendar time.

Because of the acknowledged weaknesses of studies that rely entirely on automated data (Chen et al., 1997; Mullooly et al., 1999; Verstraeten et al., 2003b), VSD researchers often conduct case-control studies to test potential relationships between vaccines and selected outcomes. The case-control studies involve a targeted set of individuals with and without the outcomes of interest. Additional data are collected through individual medical record review, patient surveys or interviews, or clinical examinations. Those additional measures provide data of considerably higher quality with respect to completeness, accuracy, and comprehensive control for potential confounding factors.

Independent external researchers who need chart-review-verified data or other primary data collection for new studies must ask the MCOs for permission to do chart reviews and provide funding for this activity. If they cannot obtain such data and want to conduct studies of new hypotheses through the data sharing program, they must rely solely on the automated data from the MCOs' administrative databases, which are now available only for events that occurred in or before 2000.

Recommendation 3.2: The committee recommends that the distinction between the annual automated VSD data (whose quality cannot always be guaranteed) available to independent external researchers through the data sharing program and the study-specific data potentially available to researchers affiliated with the NIP or

the participating MCOs be explained more clearly in the data sharing guidelines so that potential users are informed about the limitations of the data that are available through the data sharing program.

Need for Collaboration

According to the VSD contract provisions, data for events on January 1, 2001, and later remain the property of the MCOs, and the NIP and NCHS are bound by the contract restrictions. The contract provisions allow independent external researchers access only to automated data for events before January 1, 2001, for new studies. Because the quality of automated data cannot be guaranteed, the inclusion of chart-review-verified data in new vaccine safety studies improves the quality of such studies. Chart-review-verified data can be obtained only by collaborating with NIP-affiliated or MCO-affiliated researchers. Thus, it is important for independent external researchers to try to collaborate with a NIP-affiliated or MCO-affiliated researcher to produce a new, high-quality vaccine safety study with recent VSD data. The committee recognizes that data limitations may severely limit some independent external uses of the VSD and compromise the quality of VSD data in new studies by independent researchers who do not gain access to data beyond the automated datasets. The committee sees no alternative to that situation for an independent external researcher who cannot or will not collaborate with NIP-affiliated or MCO-affiliated VSD researchers, and this underscores the need for a system that supports and, to the extent feasible, ensures collaboration when requested.

There are many reasons why collaboration for the access, use, and interpretation of VSD data is necessary. The VSD is a complex database, and external researchers could benefit substantially from the knowledge and experience of researchers who have already conducted research with the VSD or similar administrative databases. By collaborating with researchers who have experience with and knowledge of the capabilities and limitations of the VSD database, external researchers with little experience in analyzing VSD data may be in a better position to use and interpret VSD findings. Chart-reviewed data can be obtained only through collaboration with the MCOs. However, NIP-affiliated or MCO-affiliated researchers that collaborate with external researchers should not attempt to censor or discourage the testing of any particular hypotheses; all types of vaccine safety hypotheses should be considered.

Because independent external researchers can use the VSD data sharing program for new studies only with data for events before 2001, the only way that such researchers can conduct new studies with all years of VSD data (in particular, data from 2001 and later) is, in effect, to collaborate with NIP-affiliated or MCO-affiliated researchers. That creates obvious hurdles for independent external researchers:

- Some independent external researchers may not want to collaborate with researchers from the NIP or one of the MCOs affiliated with the VSD;
- Even when an external researcher desires to collaborate, collaboration by its very nature cannot be forced. If there is not a willing researcher affiliated with the NIP or one of the MCOs, the venture probably will not succeed; and
- There are no mechanisms to encourage collaboration.

The committee believes that NIP-affiliated or MCO-affiliated VSD researchers should not be forced to collaborate with independent external researchers but that collaboration should be encouraged. Ensuring that someone at each MCO is responsible for facilitating collaborative relationships is one way to overcome the limitations of the VSD data sharing program for new studies that require use of data from 2001 and later. Such a person should serve as a contact person who connects interested external researchers with interested MCO-affiliated researchers; a facilitator should not necessarily be expected to also be a collaborator. The committee notes, however, that ensuring a workable system for collaboration may have implications for renegotiation of the VSD contract.

Recommendation 3.3: Because of the limitations in the data available to independent external researchers through the VSD data sharing program, the committee recommends that the NIP require the designation of a facilitator for collaboration at each MCO as a condition of the VSD contract.

Collaboration could bring other benefits to the program. Collaboration with external researchers on new vaccine safety questions and evaluation strategies could bring new ideas to the attention of NIP and MCO researchers, add to the pool of talented researchers, and bring additional resources to bear on vaccine issues. Greater collaboration also might have an independent effect on increasing mutual understanding and reducing differences in the interpretation of findings. But collaboration raises practical challenges. If intent and commitment to openness and fairness do not undergird a system of collaboration, it will fail. Barriers and unnecessary hurdles may be interpreted as efforts to suppress interpretations that are scientifically sound and supportable—a result that would take the program backward rather than forward.

Types of Collaboration

Different types of scientific collaboration are possible. The two most common types are intramural collaboration and collaboration through a multidisciplinary team. In intramural collaboration, colleagues in the same organization collaborate on the design, development, or execution of a research project. In collaboration through a multidisciplinary team, colleagues in different organizations collaborate on the design, development, or execution of a research project. For the VSD, both types of collaboration take place; most studies require a multidisciplinary approach because most VSD studies involve data from more than one MCO.

Limitations of Data Available to External Researchers for Reanalyses

The November 2004 version of the data sharing guidelines states that "external researchers who would like to perform a reanalysis of a published VSD study performed by VSD investigators may request the final dataset for the specific study they wish to re-analyze" (CDC, 2004a). When independent external researchers have access only to final datasets from particular VSD studies, they can do little more than try different computational methods or audit the originally reported statistical calculations. Provision of a final dataset cannot support a challenge of original study design features, nor does it provide the important confirmatory step of corroboration (which would require an independent study), nor does it allow for verification that the final dataset was properly prepared. Limitation to a final dataset does not allow independent researchers to reconfigure the source data for different inclusion criteria (of either variables or subjects) or different variable definitions or coding. Testing the criteria and assumptions is often an important part of a validation exercise.

Audits of studies can offer little in the way of alternative explanations of a study's findings unless it can be shown that the original study's authors made errors in the analysis of the final dataset. Likewise, new computational procedures themselves are not likely to change conclusions if the data cannot be explored to understand why different analyses yielded different conclusions. The committee believes that a modified analysis of a published VSD study can rarely address fundamental concerns about the original study if only the final dataset is provided to independent researchers.

Recommendation 3.4: To formulate alternative hypotheses or to conduct alternative analyses, researchers need to have access to information or variables that would allow the use of different inclusion and exclusion criteria, different variables for inclusion in models,

and, in general, earlier versions of a dataset that would support such restructuring. The committee believes that it is appropriate to allow independent external researchers access to such datasets and recommends that such datasets be made available through the VSD data sharing program.

Any broadening of the data files must, of course, respect needs for patient confidentiality. The committee recognizes that implementation of this recommendation probably can affect only future VSD studies because earlier versions of study datasets may not have been archived for current or completed studies.

What Can Be Accomplished Through the VSD Data Sharing Program, Given the Limitations?

The current VSD data sharing program guidelines allow external researchers to submit proposals to conduct two types of studies: new vaccine studies and reanalyses of final datasets from published VSD studies (CDC, 2004a). However, the committee finds that at least four types of studies can be done with VSD data, and some have different needs for collaboration:

- *Audit.* Involves simply a recalculation of the statistics included in a previous study report with the same final analytic dataset; collaboration is not necessary.
- *Broader reanalysis.* Involves the examination of variables or possibly changes in the individuals included in or omitted from the final dataset but does not usually involve the entire source dataset; collaboration is not necessary but could be helpful.
- *Corroboration study.* A test of the same hypothesis with a new design or study population; collaboration is necessary to gain access to all needed data.
- *Investigation of a new hypothesis.* A new study of a previously untested hypothesis; collaboration is necessary to gain access to all needed data.

Use of those four categories (there may also be borderline categories) may help to clarify the specific datasets that will be needed by researchers, depending on the intent of their studies, and may promote more appropriate expectations of the findings and conclusions that emerge. (See Table 2 for a summary of the categories.)

Recommendation 3.5: The committee recommends that the VSD data sharing guidelines reflect a more specific categorization of the

TABLE 2 VSD Research Options for Independent External Researchers

	Pre – 1/01/01 Data	Post – 1/01/01 Data
Audit	Possible; no collaboration required	Possible; no collaboration required
Broader reanalysis	Possible; no collaboration required	Possible; no collaboration required
Corroboration study	Possible; collaboration recommended to improve quality	Not possible without collaboration
Investigation of a new hypothesis	Possible; collaboration recommended to improve quality	Not possible without collaboration

types of studies that can be done with VSD data to conceptualize the full range of studies that independent external researchers may wish to conduct with the data: an audit, a broader reanalysis, a corroboration study, and an investigation of a new hypothesis.

It also will be necessary for independent external researchers to be explicit in their proposals about the purpose of their proposed analysis: if an audit or application of an alternative statistical method is intended, a final dataset may suffice; for a broader reanalysis, access to an intermediate or extended dataset, rather than the final dataset, will almost surely be necessary; and if a corroboration study or investigation of a new hypothesis is proposed, independent external researchers will need access to source data, which may require the assistance of a VSD collaborator. When collaboration is sought, the external researchers should contact a facilitator for collaboration at each MCO (see Recommendation 3.3) to pursue a collaborative research relationship with a researcher at the MCO or contact the lead staff person for the VSD data sharing program to pursue a collaborative research relationship with a NIP-affiliated researcher. That will aid access to the data, reduce the likelihood of concerns about confidentiality, and help to facilitate direct, knowledgeable reanalyses of VSD data.

SPECIFIC COMPONENTS OF THE VACCINE SAFETY DATALINK DATA SHARING PROGRAM GUIDELINES

The committee considered modifications of the VSD data sharing program guidelines needed to facilitate use of VSD data by external researchers, to ensure appropriate utilization of the data, and to protect the confidentiality of the data. The committee has used the framework of the process that independent external researchers must follow to use VSD data through the data sharing program in formulating its recommendations on specific aspects of the guidelines.

Review of Proposals

Required Proposal Elements

All four versions of the VSD data sharing program guidelines contain information about the elements that are required or suggested in proposals for accessing VSD data (CDC, 2002, 2003a, 2004a,b). The latest version of the guidelines (CDC, 2004a) provides much more detail about the required proposal elements than previous versions. The committee finds that all the information currently required in proposals is reasonable and necessary. The committee encourages the NCHS to maintain the list of required proposal elements in future revisions of the guidelines and to consider further specifying the required information for "proposed analytic strategies" (CDC, 2004a).

Evaluation Criteria

The criteria that will be used to evaluate VSD data sharing proposals are not clear. In the August 2002, October 2003, and November 2004 (CDC, 2002, 2003a, 2004a) versions of the guidelines, no specific evaluation criteria are provided for VSD proposals. The August 2002 guidelines do not mention how proposals will be evaluated (CDC, 2002). The October 2003 guidelines simply state that the NIP will determine whether external researchers' proposals are complete and whether the requested variables are available (CDC, 2003a).

In March 2004, the programmatic responsibility for the VSD data sharing program was transferred from the NIP to NCHS (CDC, 2004d). The August 2004 version of NCHS's procedures for use of its RDC states that four criteria will be used to evaluate proposals: scientific and technical feasibility of the project, availability of resources at the RDC, risk of disclosure of restricted information, and whether the proposed project is in accordance with the NCHS mission (CDC, 2004b). In the November 2004 guidelines, NCHS states that those criteria will be used for proposals that request use of NCHS data. For VSD proposals, "RDC staff will notify the external researcher whether his/her proposal is complete and whether the requested variables are available" (CDC, 2004a); no criteria for evaluation of VSD proposals are provided. The NIP and NCHS should develop, with public input, the criteria that will be used to evaluate proposals.

Recommendation 3.6: The committee recommends that there be specific evaluation criteria for VSD proposals and that interested persons have an opportunity to comment on the draft evaluation criteria before they are finalized; the evaluation criteria should be identified clearly in the VSD data sharing guidelines.

Technical Feasibility of Proposals

To ensure appropriate utilization of VSD data, the committee agrees that it is reasonable and appropriate to evaluate the technical feasibility of a proposed study. Determining whether a study can be carried out successfully with the VSD data that are available to external researchers is important for ensuring that the resources of the NIP, NCHS, the MCOs, and the researchers are not spent on studies that have no possibility of answering a proposed question. The committee emphasizes, however, that technical feasibility should be determined on the basis of stated objective criteria. The criteria that should define technical feasibility include these:

- The requested data are available in the database.
- Enough individuals are represented in the database with the exposures and outcomes of interest to study the proposed hypothesis.
- The proposed statistical tests are possible with the available data.

The criteria are not meant to exclude novel hypotheses or novel methods. If a proposed VSD study is technically feasible with the available VSD data, even if the hypotheses or methods are considered atypical, access to the data should be approved. The technical feasibility of a proposal should be determined by an independent review committee rather than by VSD program staff.

Recommendation 3.7: The committee recommends that the technical feasibility of a proposed VSD study be the primary evaluation criterion in the review of proposals submitted to the VSD data sharing program.

If study of a hypothesis is determined not to be technically feasible with the available VSD data, the committee believes that it is reasonable and appropriate for an independent review committee to deny the proposal or return it for revision. Weaknesses found during the review process should be brought to the attention of the researchers. When a proposal is denied or returned for revision, the technical feasibility determinations or other determinations that prompted the decision should be clearly and adequately described to the applicants. However, it should remain the responsibility of the researchers, not the NIP or NCHS, to ensure that the proposal is revised to meet the requirements.

Recommended Competencies

It is reasonable to expect that external researchers who wish to use VSD data have specific competencies, such as the ability to use SAS or an equivalent statistical analysis package, experience in using claims data, adequate knowledge of epidemiologic methods, and the ability to select and interpret statistical tests. The committee believes that the lack of such competencies should not in itself be a reason to deny or require revisions to a VSD proposal. If the competencies that will be helpful in analyzing VSD data appropriately are delineated, it may help external researchers (who may include consumers interested in conducting research) to gain an understanding of competencies that they may want to develop or acquire through additional consultations or collaborations in a team approach. That may save much time, effort, and frustration during the limited time that researchers have for access to the VSD data at the NCHS RDC. A list of recommended competencies should be used to assist external researchers in preparing to use VSD data at the RDC and should not be used to discourage external researchers from submitting research proposals for the VSD data sharing program.

> Recommendation 3.8: To assist independent external researchers who want to use VSD data through the data sharing program, the committee recommends that the NIP and NCHS add to the VSD data sharing program guidelines a list of recommended competencies for VSD data analysis.

Technical Assistance

Not all external researchers may want to pursue a collaborative research project with a NIP-affiliated or MCO-affiliated researcher who previously has analyzed VSD data. However, external researchers who want to conduct a VSD study independently should not expect to receive extensive technical assistance (such as advice and guidance on appropriate statistical tests, on confounders that should be considered, or on statistical analysis programs) from the NIP or NCHS in developing their proposal or using the data at the NCHS RDC. NIP and NCHS employees already have major tasks in developing and using the VSD data sharing program and should not be diverted from other required duties by requests from external researchers for extensive technical assistance.

Submission of Proposals to Institutional Review Boards at the Managed Care Organizations

The VSD could not exist without the voluntary participation of the MCOs whose members' data constitute it. By law, the MCOs are responsible for ensuring the confidentiality of their members' health information. Confidentiality protections must not be jeopardized; a single breach of confidentiality, no matter how minor, could undermine the contractual arrangements between the MCOs and the NIP and lead to the termination of cooperation and the loss of a unique resource of potentially great national value. Protecting the confidentiality of the information requires that procedures for use of the VSD be clearly stated and explained in the VSD data sharing guidelines.

Institutional Review Board Application Process for VSD Proposals

The VSD data sharing program guidelines require that independent external researchers receive approval from the IRB at each MCO whose data will be accessed. That requirement can mean that researchers must submit applications to up to nine IRBs (one of the MCO sites requires application to two IRBs) (CDC, 2004d). Each IRB has its own application formats, rules, procedures, and timelines for reviewing VSD proposals. Approvals for data access are for 1 year at a time; because IRBs work on different schedules, the first approval may expire before the last is granted.

Although previous users of the VSD data sharing program believed that the process was too burdensome (Geier and Geier, 2004), review by each participating institution is a standard element of multisite studies. IRB review processes generally take months rather than weeks in part because of the frequent need for repeated revision and clarification of proposals, and some IRBs charge fees (McNay et al., 2002). The MCO IRB approval process took about 6 months for the only group of researchers who accessed VSD data through the data sharing program (Geier and Geier, 2004), but the process included multiple revisions and clarifications; the researchers also were charged $1,500 by one of the IRBs involved in the program. IRB review is expensive in personnel time. The committee concludes that the time and costs of IRB review (among institutions that charge for IRB review) that were experienced by the previous users of the VSD (Geier and Geier, 2004) are fair and within the normal range for IRB review of various types of research proposals, given the nature of these proposals.

Burdens Caused by Multiple Institutional Review Board Applications

Even with the reasonable and customary requirements of IRBs, efforts could be made to make the IRB application process less burdensome. Independent external researchers should not be unduly hindered or delayed in accessing VSD data, so it is important that the IRB review process move quickly, without jeopardizing the careful review of provisions for protecting confidentiality. Because independent external researchers are required to gain IRB approval from multiple MCOs for any VSD study, the committee believes that in the spirit of public access and transparency, unnecessary hurdles imposed on those wishing to use the VSD data sharing program should be minimized.

Use of an IRB authorization agreement could be one way to streamline the IRB application process for independent external researchers. An IRB authorization agreement allows an institution to rely on another institution's IRB for review and continuing oversight of its human subjects research (HHS, 2002). IRB authorization agreements can be used for all human subjects research at an institution or can be limited to specific research protocols (HHS, 2002). The IRB that conducts the review reports its findings and actions to appropriate officials at the other institution. The institution that delegated its IRB review is responsible for ensuring compliance with the IRB's determinations, even though it is relying on the IRB of the other institution. For research proposals submitted through the VSD data sharing program, use of IRB authorization agreements could streamline the IRB approval process for independent external researchers by reducing the number of MCO IRB applications that must be submitted.

> **Recommendation 3.9: To facilitate use of the VSD data sharing program, the committee recommends that the NIP work with the VSD-participating MCOs to determine the feasibility of using IRB authorization agreements for VSD research proposals.**

Burdens Caused by Institutional Review Board Requirements for Reanalyses

The committee finds that the requirement for IRB approval from each MCO whose data would be examined in a reanalysis of a previously published study could be burdensome and may inhibit reanalyses. To do a reanalysis, independent external researchers are required to seek IRB approval from each MCO whose data were included in the final dataset. If one IRB denies the application, the researchers cannot conduct a true reanalysis. That potentially reduces the value of the data sharing program because there is no recourse if one IRB chooses to deny or limit access to final datasets from studies that have already been published. That a study is a reanalysis means that the MCOs' IRBs approved a previous analysis of the final dataset. The committee understands that there is a new disclosure risk in allowing different researchers access to such a dataset, but the previous approval for analysis of the dataset and rigorous confidentiality provisions in place at the RDC argue at least for expedited review of IRB applications for reanalyses.

> **Recommendation 3.10: The committee recommends that the NIP work with the MCOs participating in the VSD and America's Health Insurance Plans (the VSD contractor) to evaluate the feasibility of streamlining the IRB review process for audits or broader reanalyses in accordance with appropriate regulations.**

Use of the NCHS Research Data Center

Confidentiality Protections at the RDC

When independent external researchers access MCO data, NCHS takes extensive measures to ensure the confidentiality of individually identifiable information. When MCO-affiliated or NIP-affiliated researchers use VSD data, their employers have provisions (for example, the possibility of termination of employment) that can help to ensure that confidentiality is not violated. When independent external researchers are granted access to data, the primary way to ensure confidentiality is to protect it at the time of data analysis. For the VSD, the confidentiality protections operate through the restrictions in place at the NCHS RDC.

When independent external researchers want to use VSD data for a particular study, NCHS must prepare data files that contain only the data required by the approved proposal. Researchers must work within the physical confines of the RDC, and no electronic or hard copies of data files or documents may leave the RDC without passing disclosure limitation review (CDC, 2004a). Restrictions go beyond personal identifiers and include unique or unusual combinations of elements that might apply to few people (for example, inpatient admission of a 56-year-old man to a specific MCO on a specific date could well be used to identify a particular person). Therefore, table cells with fewer than five observations are customarily blocked by NCHS before a table leaves the RDC (CDC, 2003c), as are tables with geographic variables in any dimension, models with geographic variables as outcome variables, or case listings (CDC, 2004a).

Fair Application of Confidentiality Provisions

The committee is concerned that the restrictions placed on independent external researchers, compared with NIP-affiliated or MCO-affiliated VSD researchers, are not applied equitably. For example, independent external researchers using the VSD data sharing program are not permitted to see table cells that contain fewer than five observations (CDC, 2004a). However, internal VSD researchers have published papers in which the cells in some tables contain fewer than five observations (Verstraeten et al., 2003a). It is understandable that some additional restrictions on data access need to be in place for researchers not affiliated with one of the parties to the VSD contract, but equitable application of the confidentiality restrictions on all researchers will help to ensure public trust in the VSD data sharing program. The committee concludes that some of those concerns can be addressed by use of an independent review committee for oversight of research protocols (see Recommendation 5.3).

Enforcement of Confidentiality Provisions

Violations of the confidentiality provisions of the RDC are subject to federal law and are punishable under Title 18 of the United States Code, section 1001, by a fine of up to $10,000 or imprisonment for up to 5 years (CDC, 2004a). To help to ensure that the confidentiality of individually identifiable VSD data is not jeopardized, data requesters should be informed clearly about the penalties and about the strict sanctions for any violations of confidentiality. An understanding that there will be strict enforcement of confidentiality requirements may help to ensure that researchers take their responsibility to safeguard confidentiality very seriously.

The general rules for use of the NCHS RDC require that researchers sign the *Agreement Regarding Conditions of Access to Confidential Data in the Research Data Center of the National Center for Health Statistics* (can be found in Appendix G) (CDC, 2004a). This agreement states that:

> Deliberate violation of any of these conditions may result in cancellation of the data access agreement, and the researcher may be escorted from the premises by the duly authorized Federal protection service on duty at NCHS. The researcher may also be barred from any future use of the RDC upon review and determination by the Director of NCHS that this is necessary to protect the integrity and confidentiality of the RDC.

On the basis of the information that is included for the project-specific requirements for the VSD (CDC, 2004a), it is not clear whether that provision applies to use of VSD data at the RDC or only to use of NCHS data at the RDC.

Recommendation 3.11: Because the confidentiality concerns are integral to the continuation of the VSD, the committee recommends that NCHS in conjunction with the MCOs develop policies and pro-

cedures to address confidentiality violations of VSD data and that they be clearly described in the VSD data sharing program guidelines and the agreements that external researchers must sign before using the RDC.

Costs for Use of the RDC

Most researchers in any field of health or medicine must obtain grant or contract funding to pay the costs of doing research, including the cost of access to data. As with other databases, the VSD data holder (NCHS) incurs costs (primarily personnel costs) when it allows independent external researchers access to the VSD database. Submission of a proposal generates personnel costs to NCHS for its review and follow-up. The committee believes that the costs to external researchers for use of the VSD are reasonable, compared with the costs for using other data enclaves. NCHS should not be expected to cover the costs of these activities out of its current funding, which is allocated for other activities. It is reasonable to expect independent external researchers who want to use VSD data to acquire or provide funding to support their research.

> **Recommendation 3.12:** The committee concludes that it is reasonable to expect researchers who request access to VSD data to have their own funding and it therefore recommends that RDC costs not be waived for independent external researchers.

Reporting Objectives, Methods, and Results

Sharing information about any studies or analyses done with VSD data can have many benefits. First, providing information about the objectives, methods, and results of studies promotes transparency, and greater transparency can enhance public trust (McComas, 2004a,b). Sharing details about the methods used for particular studies can assist other researchers who are interested in pursuing a reanalysis or a corroboration of a study with a different database.

In the next chapter, the committee describes why it is important to share as much programmatic information as possible about current and completed VSD studies. The committee discusses how the NIP should share information about any studies conducted by NIP-affiliated or MCO-affiliated researchers. Likewise, the committee finds that the need for transparency should also apply to independent external researchers who use VSD data. If NIP-affiliated and MCO-affiliated researchers will be asked to share their research protocols, fairness and transparency require that external researchers do the same.

As stewards of the data, the NIP and NCHS should know how VSD data are being used. One way is to ensure that the NIP and NCHS have standardized information on each study conducted through the VSD data sharing program by requiring independent external researchers to provide specific information on any studies conducted through the program. Requiring standardized, specific information from users of the data sharing program and standardized research protocols from internal VSD researchers will leave all VSD researchers subject to similar information-sharing requirements.

> **Recommendation 3.13: The committee recommends that, as a condition of accessing VSD data, all independent external researchers that use the VSD data sharing program be required to submit a report to the NIP (with a copy to NCHS) within a reasonable time (to be determined by the NIP) on the status of their study, the type of study conducted (an audit, a broader reanalysis, a corroboration study, or an investigation of a new hypothesis), the results obtained, and their planned further activities. The reports should be made public by the NIP and should be easily accessible.**

Correspondingly, when researchers are preparing a public release of findings from data that were accessed through the VSD data sharing program (for example, in a presentation at a conference or meeting or in a journal article), the committee finds it reasonable to expect that the data steward (the NIP and NCHS) will be notified of the release of the findings within a reasonable time. When the findings are released, there may be questions about the benefits and limitations of the database, the study population, and the analyses that are appropriate given the structure of the database. The data steward may be called on to explain how the findings presented in the publication or presentation support or contradict other findings derived from the same database. Being able to provide an explanation for how the findings compare with other findings derived from the database can help to give the public the appropriate context for understanding the new findings. It is therefore appropriate for the data steward to have an opportunity to prepare for such questions. However, the committee believes that a requirement for advance notification of the release of findings should not be used as an opportunity to censor findings or to release similar findings in advance of the researchers' planned release; any evidence to the contrary should be reviewed by an independent review committee.

> **Recommendation 3.14: The committee recommends that, as a condition of accessing VSD data, all independent external researchers that use the VSD data sharing program be required to submit to the NIP (with a copy to NCHS) a copy of a manuscript intended for**

publication at least 30 days before submission to a journal or other print or electronic media. Copies of presentations to be delivered at conferences or meetings that are open to the public or that have media coverage should also be submitted to the NIP and NCHS at least 15 days before presentation.

Failure to comply with either of those reporting requirements could be grounds for NCHS to deny future access to VSD data through the data sharing program.

Creation of a Basic Analytic File

The VSD is a complex database, and generally only sophisticated users will be able to master use of its data files. The NIP and NCHS may want to explore the creation of a basic analytic file that could be used to answer many questions of interest to external researchers. Such a data file would not replace all specific data files that might be requested by independent external researchers for particular studies, but it could serve as a useful resource for many researchers to develop and refine hypotheses and to begin understanding how to use the VSD files in the RDC.

The committee recognizes that the creation of such a data file, with full protections of confidentiality, would require considerable time and effort. The cost of such a resource should be assessed and made publicly available so that Congress and other stakeholders would have the information necessary to make an informed decision regarding a possible investment of public funds. The creation of such a data file should be pursued only if additional funds are made available for the purpose. The availability of a cleaned, standard analytic file to a variety of researchers could help to foster appropriate use of the dataset by external researchers and to reduce the burden on both NCHS and researchers who want to analyze VSD data.

4

The Vaccine Safety Datalink Research Process and the Release of Preliminary Findings

REVIEW OF ITERATIVE ANALYSIS APPROACHES USED FOR VACCINE SAFETY DATALINK STUDIES

In its charge, the committee was asked to "review the iterative approaches to conducting analysis that are characteristics of studies using the complex, automated Vaccine Safety Datalink (VSD) system. Examples of recent studies to be examined are a completed screening study on thimerosal and vaccines (Verstraeten et al., 2003a) and cohort studies on asthma." The studies by DeStefano et al. (2002) and by Verstraeten et al. (2003a) are reviewed below.

Childhood Vaccinations and Risk of Asthma

The 2002 study by DeStefano and colleagues evaluated a suggested association between the risk of asthma and childhood vaccines by studying a retrospective cohort. The researchers found no association between asthma and diptheria-tetanus-pertussis vaccine, oral polio vaccine, or measles-mumps-rubella vaccine. They found weak associations of asthma with *Haemophilus influenzae* type b vaccine and Hepatitis B vaccine, which the authors attributed partially to a bias in health care utilization or information bias (for example, they could not verify that a child who according to the medical record was unvaccinated was not accessing health care elsewhere) (DeStefano et al., 2002).

Review of Timeline

In January 1997, a proposal on asthma studies was put forward by a researcher at the Centers for Disease Control and Prevention (CDC), and a working group consisting of interested investigators from the VSD, managed care organizations (MCOs), and CDC was established to conduct such studies.[1] In fall 1997, a paper by Kemp and colleagues (Kemp et al., 1997) suggested an association between whole-cell pertussis vaccine and asthma. Around that time, several articles were published on the hygiene hypothesis (Mawson, 2001), which posits that some infections in infancy or early childhood may protect against asthma or other allergic conditions. That raised the idea that vaccines, by preventing the infections, may increase the risk of asthma. The National Immunization Program (NIP) decided that this topic should be addressed by using VSD data, so NIP-affiliated VSD researchers conducted a pilot study in 1998 (DeStefano, 2004).

The study team was able to conduct data-quality and data-assurance checks of the electronic data and perform chart review on a sample of about 5% of the VSD population. The study team used that 5% sample to do the analyses. The analyses were presented at a meeting of VSD investigators in June 1998 and at the Interscience Conference on Antimicrobial Agents and Chemotherapy (ICAAC) in September 1998. The researchers determined that even though they had reviewed the patient charts, there was uncertainty about the MCO enrollment status of children; some were enrolled from birth, and others were enrolled when they were 2 or 3 years old. The researchers could not determine with certainty the patients' vaccine histories before they were enrolled in the MCO. From the pilot study, the researchers learned that the data were not complete enough to be sure that the children who did not have vaccinations in their records were not vaccinated (DeStefano, 2004).

The researchers revised their study on the basis of what they had learned and restricted the data analysis to children born as MCO members to obtain a complete vaccination history. The initial findings from the new analysis were presented at the May 1999 meeting of VSD investigators. There was still some concern about the validity of vaccination status, and to account for it, the researchers conducted a subanalysis of children who had at least some indication of using the MCO for health care. The findings of the analysis were presented at the International Conference on Pharmacoepidemiology in August 1999 and at the September 1999

---

[1]Personal communication, F. DeStefano, NIP, February 10, 2005.

ICAAC. The findings were the same as the main results in the final paper (DeStefano, 2004).

The publication of the manuscript took over 3 years (January 1999-June 2002). The first draft was completed in January 1999, and it was cleared by CDC and ready for submission to a scientific journal by October 2000 (the paper was not accepted by the first journal and was submitted to a second journal in May 2001) (DeStefano, 2004). The second journal also did not accept the submission, so it was sent to a third journal (*Journal of Pediatric Infectious Disease*) in August 2001, was accepted in February 2002, and published in June 2002 (DeStefano, 2004; DeStefano et al., 2002).

Safety of Thimerosal-Containing Vaccines: A Two-Phase Study of Computerized MCO Databases

The 2003 study by Verstraeten and colleagues explored possible associations between thimerosal (a preservative that contains ethylmercury) in vaccines and neurodevelopmental disorders. The study was intended to be an initial screen of possible associations; a detailed study would be planned if any associations were identified (DeStefano, 2004). The final results based on one MCO's data indicated that cumulative exposure to thimerosal at the age of 3 months resulted in a significant association with tics (Verstraeten et al., 2003a). In data from a second MCO, an increased risk of language delay was associated with cumulative exposure at the ages of 3 months and 7 months (DeStefano, 2004). Those findings could not be replicated with data from a third, comparable MCO. None of the analyses showed a significant increase in risk of attention deficit hyperactivity disorder (ADHD) or autism (DeStefano, 2004).

Review of Timeline

The concern about thimerosal-containing vaccines and possible health effects received a lot of attention in summer 1999 when a joint Public Health Service (PHS) and American Academy of Pediatrics statement recommended reduction or elimination of thimerosal in vaccines as a precautionary measure (CDC, 1999b). That was suggested because it had been determined that with some vaccination schedules at that time, a child could have exceeded the Environmental Protection Agency's guidelines for exposure to methylmercury. In August 1999, a National Vaccine Advisory Committee meeting was convened at the National Institutes of Health (NIH) to review the research then available on the question and to recommend additional research (Egan, 2000). After the meeting, a working group of the PHS, including some external experts, was established to develop ideas for research projects that could begin to evaluate if there may have been adverse effects from thimerosal-containing vaccines.[2] One of the proposed projects was to use the VSD to explore possible associations between thimerosal and neurodevelopmental disorders. The neurologic conditions that potentially could be caused by thimerosal were not clear, so the initial analysis was used as a screening tool (DeStefano, 2004).

In fall 1999, the thimerosal working group deemed the VSD project to have high priority. The protocol for the study was developed in collaboration with the working group and the VSD principal investigators. In late fall and early winter 1999, preliminary analyses were conducted. From late February to April 2000, the analyses and preliminary findings began to be discussed among the VSD investigators. Suggestions were made on how to revise the analysis. At the April 2000 meeting of VSD investigators, the analysis had progressed to a point where there were indications of possible associations with speech or language delay and some possible associations with ADHD. The VSD investigators alerted NIP leadership of their results and sought input on how to proceed (DeStefano, 2004).

In April 2000, the lead study author presented preliminary findings at the annual Epidemic Intelligence Service conference. On April 27, 2000, the researchers briefed the CDC associate director of science on the results. It was suggested that the researchers convene a review panel of CDC scientists outside the NIP. The meeting took place in May 2000; it was determined that the evidence of an association was weak but that the results should be explored further (DeStefano, 2004). At a different May 2000 meeting with the CDC scientific review panel, a recommendation was made to try to replicate the findings in an independent dataset. The researchers conducted the replication with data from Harvard Pilgrim MCO (DeStefano, 2004).

In early June 2000, an external expert review group was convened at Simpsonwood Conference and Retreat Center (Simpsonwood Transcript, 2000). That group also determined that the evidence was weak but should be explored further along several lines of inquiry, including attempted replication with an independent database. In June 2000, the results were presented to the Advisory Committee on Immunization Practices, including findings from the third MCO (the independent database). In that third database, the researchers did not replicate findings of any of the associations seen in data from the two VSD MCOs (DeStefano, 2004). In August 2000, the findings were presented to the World Health Organization Global Vaccine Advisory Committee (GVAC). The GVAC recommended that

---

[2]Personal communication, F. DeStefano, NIP, February 10, 2005.

a similar study be done in the United Kingdom with the General Practice Research Database. In July 2001, the researchers presented updated preliminary findings to the Institute of Medicine Committee on Immunization Safety Review (Verstraeten, 2001). The updated results were fairly similar to those of earlier analyses; there were still some indications of association with speech or language delay and perhaps with attention problems (DeStefano, 2004).

The principal researcher on the thimerosal study left CDC in July 2001, but in December 2000, before he left, he wrote a first draft of a manuscript on the study and submitted it for CDC clearance (DeStefano, 2004). Because many of the researchers had moved on to other studies, it took over a year for the manuscript to be completed. Additional follow-up data became available, and improved ideas for addressing concerns about healthcare-seeking bias emerged (DeStefano, 2004).

In October 2002, the revised manuscript was submitted for CDC clearance. It was cleared by December 2002.[3] The manuscript was also submitted to the first journal for publication in that month. In May 2003, it was accepted by the second journal it was submitted to (*Pediatrics*), pending revision. The researchers revised it and resubmitted it in June. It was accepted in July, and published in November 2003 (DeStefano, 2004; Verstraeten et al., 2003a).

VACCINE SAFETY DATALINK RESEARCH PLAN

The VSD is the only population-based resource in the nation that has sufficient sample size to address possible concerns about rare adverse effects of vaccines. The VSD is an important national resource. As a resource, however, rather than a study, its value depends primarily on the nature and extent of its use. The investigators who have conducted studies with it have been almost exclusively those who are also responsible for its funding, creation, development, or maintenance. Within that community of researchers, opportunities to propose and lead studies have been created and prioritized, systems for conducting studies have been developed, and funding has been allocated.

For researchers outside the VSD research network, the opportunities and support for use of this resource have been, at best, unclear and narrow. Similarly, there appear to be few opportunities for individuals or parties outside of the NIP or the VSD MCOs to have direct input into research priorities and the allocation of resources. Finally, the public has not been routinely informed about the status and ultimate findings of research efforts undertaken with the VSD.

---

[3]Personal communication, F. DeStefano, NIP, February 10, 2005.

Those apparent shortcomings arise in part from the changing public expectations about data sharing, policy-making, and public access to information. Because the NIP is responsible for all those roles as they are related to vaccine safety data, the confluence of increasing expectations brings considerable pressure to bear on the NIP. Because the mission of the NIP is perceived to be contradictory (promoting vaccines and assessing their safety), it is all the more incumbent on the VSD to define a process whereby interested parties may give voice to their concerns, the priorities and allocations of resources are determined in open discussion, and accountability is established.

Recommendation 4.1: To enhance the value of the VSD, to improve the credibility of results derived from it, and to support CDC's role in assessing vaccine safety, the committee recommends that the NIP develop an annual VSD research plan. The plan should define the priorities for new studies and support of current studies. The annual VSD research plan should be made public. Material deviations from the plan should be identified and be publicly available.

Public Input on VSD Research Plan

The annual VSD research plan should be developed with broad input from interested parties. Many individuals and agencies have a stake in VSD activities and findings, some with conflicting needs and agendas. It is appropriate for all of them to understand and have input into the identification and ranking of new research initiatives that will use the VSD.

Scientific organizations have recognized the importance of public input in establishing priorities for research. To establish a process for gathering public input on VSD research priorities, NIP could learn from the activities of those organizations and the models they have used to involve the public in the research priority-setting process. The NIH, for example, has a Council of Public Representatives (COPR), which regularly provides advice to the director of NIH on issues related to public participation in NIH activities, outreach efforts, and other matters of public interest (NIH, 2005a). A recent report by COPR identified principles and recommendations to improve public input and transparency in the NIH research priority-setting process (COPR and NIH, 2004). Several of the principles identified in that report (for example, fostering two-way communication on an individual and community level, ensuring that senior decision-makers receive and fully consider public input, and partnering with local communities, grassroots organizations, and local leaders) could inform future VSD research activities.

Set-Aside of VSD Funding for Collaborative Projects

The principal investigators at the VSD MCOs and key senior investigators at the MCOs and CDC make decisions about which studies to undertake with VSD funds.[4] Only researchers affiliated with the NIP or the MCOs have an opportunity to propose VSD studies. Substantial federal funds are used to support the VSD infrastructure and specific VSD studies. The committee finds it reasonable for the public to expect that some portion of the contract funding will be made available to support meritorious research proposals by researchers not affiliated with the NIP or the VSD MCOs.

Recommendation 4.2: To support greater use of the VSD and to promote opportunities for collaborative work outside the existing community of VSD researchers, the committee recommends that the annual VSD research plan include provisions for allocating some existing funds, on a competitive basis, to external researchers interested in conducting collaborative work with VSD data.

Proposals should be reviewed by an independent committee that has expertise in vaccines, immunology, epidemiology, statistics, and research with administrative databases. Review should consider scientific merit, feasibility, innovative use of the VSD, and the potential to interest others in its use.

If one of the identified high-priority research subjects interests external researchers, they should have the opportunity to compete for VSD research funds. The committee believes that all public funds for VSD research should be allocated according to the priorities established through the public process. However, the committee's recommendations do not preclude submission by independent external researchers of a VSD research proposal on any hypothesis that is technically feasible; if the hypothesis is not considered to have high-priority for VSD research funds, the researchers would have to obtain other funding to conduct the study.

Detailed Documentation of Research Protocols by Internal VSD Researchers

Research proposals are generated before a study starts to describe the proposed research hypothesis, outline the research methods that will be used, identify the staff that will work on the study, and estimate a budget for the study. Detailed research protocols generally are developed after a research proposal is approved but before the study commences and in-

---

[4]Personal communication, F. DeStefano, NIP, February 10, 2005.

clude specific information about how each step in the study process will be accomplished (such as all the variables that will be included in the analyses, a detailed description of the approach to data analysis, the specific analyses and statistical tests that will be done, and the confounders that will be considered). In contrast with the more general description of research methods included in research proposals, research protocols include detailed specifications of research methods for all phases of the study.

Detailed documentation of research protocols, analysis decisions, and deviations from protocols is important for ensuring the integrity of the scientific process and specifically for ensuring public confidence in the integrity of VSD studies conducted by NIP-affiliated and MCO-affiliated VSD researchers. Thorough documentation and archiving of all study methods and analysis decisions can be considered the equivalent of keeping good laboratory notebooks. If an audit or a reanalysis of a study by an internal VSD researcher ever is conducted, thorough documentation of methods will insulate the original investigator from unwarranted criticism of the research methods used and aid the later researcher in conducting an audit or reanalysis. Having detailed research protocols for all VSD studies conducted by NIP-affiliated and MCO-affiliated researchers will support transparency of the VSD research program. Increasing the rigor with which such studies are documented and conducted will enhance public trust in findings from the VSD.

> **Recommendation 4.3: The committee recommends that detailed research protocols for each study conducted by an internal VSD researcher be developed, peer-reviewed, and archived. Each protocol should include well-specified definitions of the study population, exposures, and cases; detailed analytic plans; sample size requirements; and study timelines. Data collection forms, procedures, data and analysis files, programming code, and database versions should be documented, cataloged, and archived for a period of at least 7 years after completion of a study.**

SHARING VACCINE SAFETY DATALINK PROGRAM INFORMATION

At its meetings, the committee heard requests for more information about VSD studies and the VSD data sharing program (Bernard, 2004; Fisher, 2004a). Transparency through the provision of more information can help to ease concerns about the implementation of the VSD program. The VSD is supported by public funds, and the committee finds it reasonable to expect that as much study-specific and programmatic information as possible be shared with the public without jeopardizing confidentiality or researchers' ability to publish their work.

Sharing Information About Current and Completed Studies

Sharing information about current and completed studies is an important part of promoting transparency. The NIP has shared information about published VSD studies, but the committee concludes that it is just as important to share information about current and completed studies that are not yet published. The list of VSD publications and presentations on the NIP Web site has not been updated since December 2000 (CDC, 2000). The committee encourages the NIP to update the list often and on a fixed schedule so that the public can be assured that all studies that have been done with VSD data are disclosed quickly. Only when information about how VSD resources are being allocated is openly shared can there be public accountability for the VSD research studies that are being pursued.

A VSD research clearinghouse like that established for the California Health Interview Survey (CHIS) (CHIS, 2003) could help to promote collaboration and information-sharing among new and experienced VSD researchers. The CHIS Research Clearinghouse provides information about studies that have been completed or are in progress (CHIS, 2003), and a mailing list is used to distribute the latest news and information about CHIS to interested persons—an example of another activity that the NIP could emulate to promote transparency of VSD activities. Providing information about studies that are in progress is an important way to promote credibility, trust, and transparency between the NIP and members of the public who are concerned about vaccine safety. Such a research clearinghouse would also constitute a mechanism for promoting collaboration in that external researchers who are interested in conducting studies with VSD data could more easily identify experienced VSD researchers with whom they might collaborate.

> **Recommendation 4.4: To promote collaboration and information-sharing, the committee recommends that the NIP update and improve its list of publications and presentations by establishing a VSD research clearinghouse that provides on a timely basis status reports, study findings, and conclusions for current and completed VSD studies.**

Sharing Information About Utilization of the VSD Data Sharing Program

Transparency is an important part of ensuring public trust and confidence in the VSD. Considering that the VSD data sharing program demands could increase in the future, releasing information to the public on the use of the program (such as number and types of proposals submitted, disposition of each proposal, and timelines of notifications to researchers) could promote transparency and help to foster public trust. If the public is confident that there is a transparent, standardized process for documenting the status of proposals and that information about use of the VSD data sharing program is made known on a regular schedule, there may be less concern and suspicion about the processes that the NIP and NCHS use to implement the data sharing program.

Recommendation 4.5: The committee recommends that the NIP and NCHS release publicly the procedures that will be used for record-keeping of VSD data sharing program documents and update the status of the program regularly.

Such information could be made available electronically (for example, on the NIP or NCHS Web site) to balance the public's need for information with the administrative burden on NIP and NCHS staff. The NIP Web site may be an effective place to provide such information, especially considering that the site recently has been recognized by the World Health Organization as a vaccine safety Web site that meets essential information practices criteria (WHO, 2005).

THE ROLE OF PEER REVIEW

Peer review of completed manuscripts is an important component of the scientific process. Regardless of the type of researcher, the data being used, or the sponsor of the research, all research findings should go through peer review before being considered scientifically valid. Whereas external peer-review processes are normally used before findings are released in a peer-reviewed journal, solely internal peer-review processes may be used when questions arise about the advisability of releasing preliminary findings. Independent external peer-review processes offer the greatest confidence in the accuracy and validity of study findings. When external peer review is not possible (for example, in the case of release of preliminary findings with an urgent public health impact or through a mechanism other than a peer-reviewed journal), all findings that will be released should at least go through an extensive internal peer-review process.

The Peer-Review Process for Intramural Research at CDC

Research conducted by federal scientists goes through a slightly different peer-review process from that of research conducted by academic scientists. Because intramural research conducted by federal employees is conducted as part of the employees' regular duties, the employer (the federal government) requires that there be additional layers of review.

The NIP has described two processes that are used for review of intramural research conducted by NIP employees. The choice depends on whether the public health concern is considered routine or nonroutine. For routine public health concerns, the process that the NIP uses consists of (Bernier, 2004b):

1. Presentations at scientific meetings (considered work in progress)
2. Internal peer review and clearance
3. External peer review prior to publication (confidential)
4. Publication in journal
5. Sharing of final dataset for published study

For nonroutine public health concerns, the process that NIP uses consists of (Bernier, 2004b):

1. Consultations with internal scientists
2. Consultations with external scientists, including those from the vaccine industry
3. Presentations to standing advisory committees for policy recommendations
4. Communication with the public
5. Release of presented findings in summary form
6. Presentations at scientific meetings
7. Internal peer review and clearance
8. External peer review (confidential)
9. Publication in journal
10. Sharing of final dataset in published study

The delineation of the two processes leads to several questions: At what point in the research process is a determination made about whether the research topic is routine or nonroutine, and who makes the decision? What are the criteria for deciding whether a topic being investigated is routine or nonroutine? Because it may be difficult to distinguish between a routine and a nonroutine public health concern, should there be a single, standardized peer-review process? Could the validity of findings from work treated as a routine public health concern be questioned if it eventually has an important public health impact, since the findings did not have the intense internal peer review of the abbreviated process? Such questions could affect the perceived reliability and credibility of findings based on VSD data that are released by NIP-affiliated VSD researchers.

RELEASE OF PRELIMINARY FINDINGS

Standards of Practice for Preliminary Findings

To discuss whether, when, and how to release and share preliminary findings with others, it is necessary first to have a common understanding of what is meant by the term *preliminary findings*. For purposes of this report, *preliminary findings* refers to results or summaries and associated conclusions that are based on incomplete data or incomplete analyses. Because data are incorporated into the VSD database annually, concerns about preliminary findings affecting continual data accrual are not applicable here.

The question of the release of preliminary findings based on VSD data has an additional layer of complexity related to the multistage process that is used to test a hypothesis. In the VSD setting, *preliminary findings* may refer to results of the first-level analyses (based on automated data) or to results of incomplete analyses or incomplete data in second-level (case-control) studies.

Preliminary Findings Because of Incomplete Data

Data may be incomplete because the expected data have not all been collected, validated, or otherwise processed for analysis. In some literature, particularly that related to clinical trials, *interim findings* or *preliminary findings* refers to analyses of incomplete data that are expected to be repeated as data accumulate. In such circumstances, the statistical issues of multiple analyses of interim data have been examined, and methods for controlling false-positive error rates have been developed (DeMets, 2004). Repeated analyses of findings do not appear to be germane to the part of the committee's charge on releasing preliminary findings, because these studies are not typically designed to incorporate additional data over time as events accumulate.

Preliminary Findings Because of Incomplete Analyses

Even with complete data, analyses may be incomplete because some protocol-specified analyses have not been conducted. Analyses of observational data usually progress along the following lines. Early in the process, univariate distributions and simple correlations or other estimates of bivariate associations between some exposure and the outcomes of interest are calculated. If there is evidence of a relationship, increasingly sophisticated analytic approaches are used in an attempt to determine whether the associations could be attributed to other factors. Because of the inherent limitations of observational studies, the later analyses are designed to eliminate alternative explanations for the association, and to increase confidence in the strength of any remaining relationship. Only when an association persists despite every attempt to explain it away can a conclusion be drawn that a cause-effect relationship exists. The simple correlations or odds ratios first calculated would be considered preliminary findings. Normally, such first-level findings are provided in publications only in the context of the complete analyses on which conclusions are based.

Preliminary Data Compared with Preliminary Findings

The difference between *preliminary data* and *preliminary findings* must also be understood. At the committee's October 2004 meeting, representatives of the NIP described how the NIP conceptualizes *preliminary data* compared with *preliminary findings*. In the context of the VSD, the NIP defines *data* as "the underlying elements of information that lead to findings but are not the findings per se. They permit analyses or reanalyses" (Bernier, 2004b). It describes *preliminary data* as "the underlying elements of information of a study or investigation which are still incomplete or subject to change" (Bernier, 2004b). In contrast, the NIP defines *preliminary findings* as "initial results obtained from investigations or studies often expressed in summary statements or summary-like form such as tables or graphs. These results are incomplete and subject to change prior to peer-reviewed publication" (Bernier, 2004b). As those terms are related to the VSD, the committee uses the NIP's distinction between *preliminary data* and *preliminary findings*. However, the committee argues that the term *preliminary* should be used slightly differently.

Should There Ever Be Preliminary Findings?

When researchers examine study data for accuracy, perform initial analyses of them, and analyze the effect of confounding factors, their findings should be described as preliminary. When findings are considered valid enough to share with external groups (even if by invitation and limited) or to be the basis of a policy decision, the findings should not be characterized as preliminary, even if other findings or reports will be released later. Only expectations of additional data or additional revelations from further analyses should cause findings to be designated as preliminary. The committee believes that *preliminary* should be used only when there is an appreciable likelihood of a material change.

Although the committee argues for limited use of *preliminary findings* in the future, for the sake of clarity and adherence to the committee's charge it uses the NIP's conceptualization of *preliminary findings* in discussing findings, conclusions, and recommendations in this report.

The Role of Peer Review in the Release of Preliminary Findings

Conducting scientific research can be a long and slow process. From the time that a research study is proposed, it can take many months or years to conduct the research, analyze the results, draft a manuscript, have the manuscript reviewed by peers, and finally have the research results published. Data analysis typically begins with simple data summaries and simple analyses that progress to more sophisticated analyses and refinements. Associations and relative risks often appear, diminish, or vanish when additional causal factors are considered in the increasingly detailed analyses. Repeated looks at the data are often required to make sure that results are robust and reliable.

Advice and feedback from colleagues during study analyses are normal parts of the scientific process. When findings are deemed important enough to be the basis of a policy decision or to be communicated to the public, extensive and independent peer review is necessary.

Solely internal peer-review processes may be needed when preliminary findings could have a substantial impact on public health. The need to release preliminary findings rapidly may force a decision to limit peer review to peers inside the federal government; if so, the internal peer review should be as extensive as possible. The committee recognizes that an extensive, independent, external peer review may be even more necessary in such a situation, because potentially influential preliminary findings may be based on a small number of cases or on incomplete analyses. In such situations, purely internal review should be followed by external review on an expedited schedule.

In the case of the VSD, however, the committee finds that because the data are incorporated into the VSD data files annually rather than continually, there will rarely be situations in which preliminary findings are so urgent that they cannot undergo independent external peer review. Preliminary findings from true surveillance systems may yield quickly emerging findings, but this will rarely be the case with findings from the VSD. If the NIP determines that preliminary findings about potential vaccine-related risks should be communicated to the public, the peer-review process may be abbreviated, but it should not be less rigorous.

Recommendation 4.6: The committee recommends that in nearly all situations preliminary findings from the VSD be subject to independent external peer review before being communicated to the public or used as the basis of a policy decision. When CDC determines that purely internal peer review is necessary before release, external peer review should be undertaken as soon as possible.

Peer review of findings that are the basis of a vaccine safety-related policy decision should always be linked to the policy role of the NIP. The committee believes that there should be external peer review of any preliminary findings that the NIP uses as the basis of or to support a policy decision, although the external review need not be done in the traditional way. Novel approaches, such as standing committees of external reviewers or convening of reviewers by conference call, could be explored as mechanisms for obtaining independent external review.

Preliminary findings that could have an impact on public health may need to be released quickly, but the committee believes that the possibility of releasing findings through an expedited process at a peer-reviewed journal should not be dismissed outright. Many journals are able to obtain rapid peer review and release articles in electronic format on an expedited basis. The committee believes that releasing preliminary findings through an expedited process at a peer-reviewed journal should always be seen as preferable to releasing preliminary findings through a solely internal peer-review process.

Concerns About Releasing Preliminary Findings

Using the NIP's conceptualization of *preliminary findings*, the committee finds that various concerns arise in the release of preliminary findings. Most important is the need for careful balance of the needs and rights of the public to be kept informed, the added costs of satisfying those needs and rights, and the risk of unnecessary alarm or unwarranted complacency if interpretations change. The committee's deliberations about the release of preliminary findings have been guided by the need for balance of costs, risk, and benefits.

Need for Scientific Exchange

The scientific process is characterized by exchange of information, response, and revision among colleagues. That process helps to ensure that scientific results are valid and account for all possible confounding factors. During the process, preliminary findings may be shared among colleagues.

Some of the process of scientific exchange occurs outside the public context. Preliminary findings should rarely be exchanged publicly, because early interpretations are often wrong and there is scientific value in having peers review methods and analyses for rigor and accuracy. Routinely releasing preliminary findings can have an adverse effect on the broader peer-review process by seeming to condone the release of preliminary findings before they have been reviewed by peers.

Distinction Between Signals and Noise

Evidence of relationships or of a lack of relationships—signals—in scientific data is always subject to the possibility of bias and randomness—noise. The smaller the signal in relation to the noise, the greater the difficulty of interpretation and the greater the likelihood of erroneous conclusions. In scientific research, especially when data are examined iteratively, it can be difficult to determine when the results of data analysis indicate a true signal of a risk as opposed to noise. The likelihood that a conclusion is inaccurate is greater—sometimes much greater—when it is based on preliminary or interim data than when it is based on a full dataset. In summary, preliminary findings, as the committee defines them, are meant to push the envelope and are expected to be found wrong in many situations; otherwise, there would be no reason to try to improve the analysis and interpretation of the data.

Consequences When Published Findings Differ from Preliminary Findings

When final interpretations of a scientific study differ substantially from preliminary findings that are already in the public domain, there is an obvious need to explain and justify the changes. That can be a healthy part of the scientific process, but it can undermine the credibility of a study among persons who do not have a full understanding of how the scientific process works. When a policy decision is based on preliminary findings and later published findings indicate a risk that is different from the risk that influenced a policy decision, the changes may create a particularly serious problem. Such a situation can undermine not only the particular study but also the policy as a whole if the public begins to question the credibility of all the data that served as the basis of the policy. Ultimately, routine and widespread dissemination of preliminary results can sometimes undermine public trust if preliminary conclusions fail verification and are changed (Weijer, 2004).

Public Health Impact of Releasing Preliminary Findings

The decision to release preliminary findings should mean that someone deemed the findings to be important for the health of the public and that urgent notice to the public is needed. Accordingly, it can be expected—and indeed intended—that knowledge of the findings will change policy or the behavior of some segments of the public (such as consumers, health care practitioners, and researchers studying similar issues). The acknowledgment that findings can cause behavior change in some way emphasizes the importance of ensuring that preliminary findings represent a true signal and not just data noise. It can be difficult to change established health behaviors (McCall, 2003), and this underscores the importance of minimizing the likelihood that final results will support a different conclusion from preliminary results. In a larger scientific context (beyond the VSD), releasing preliminary findings can affect future data collection. That can confound final results and undermine the legitimacy of a study's conclusions.

Whenever a decision to release preliminary findings is contemplated, the risks, costs, and benefits related to early disclosure of findings compared with delayed disclosure of findings must be examined and weighed (Ball et al., 1998; Dittmann, 2001; Slovic, 1987). When releasing preliminary findings, it is important to communicate the risk properly and in a way that protects the credibility of the source so that the public can trust the findings and base appropriate health decisions on them (McComas and Trumbo, 2001). When contemplating the release of preliminary findings about vaccines, it is important to consider the effect of interrupting immunization programs, the probable size of true and perceived risks and the likelihood of unknown risks, and the risk of vaccine-preventable diseases compared with the risk reduction that could be achieved through immunization (Dittmann, 2001). Such an approach would have added benefits the next time results are released.

When to Release Preliminary Findings

Despite those concerns, in various situations it is appropriate to release preliminary findings about potential vaccine-related risks based on VSD data. In the case of the thimerosal screening analysis (Verstraeten et al., 2003a), some people retrospectively questioned the decision process used by the NIP to determine whether, when, and how to share preliminary findings with others (Bernard, 2004). The NIP did not use a formal decision mechanism to guide the release of VSD preliminary findings to others.

Retrospective assessments of the appropriateness of such decisions can offer lessons for similar situations in the future, but they do not directly provide guidance for making such decisions. That underscores the need to define a priori the conditions governing whether, when, and how to share preliminary VSD findings about potential vaccine-related risks with other scientists, the public, and policy-makers.

Release of Preliminary Findings When Shared with Others

The NIP should expect, of course, that a public release to one group will soon, and appropriately, spread to others, and the risks and costs related to selective release are powerful arguments against selective release. However, a public release should not be confused with consultations with particularly knowledgeable scientists providing peer review or the equivalent.

One of the conditions that should determine when preliminary findings are shared with the public is the process used to share the findings with other scientists. It is reasonable to expect that preliminary findings will be shared among researchers affiliated with the NIP and the MCOs and among federal employees without having to be shared with the public; this is part of the normal peer-review process for ensuring the rigor and validity of research. However, with respect to sharing preliminary findings in broader venues (for example, in presentations at scientific meetings and in meetings that involve people who do not have a role in scientific peer review), the committee believes that no members of the public have a greater right to knowledge than others. That all members of the general public should have equal access to information from the federal government is a vital component of the Federal Advisory Committee Act, the Government in the Sunshine Act, and the Freedom of Information Act.

> **Recommendation 4.7:** The committee recommends that preliminary findings from VSD data be shared with the public whenever the findings are presented to anyone *other than* collaborators in the research, federal employees responsible for research activities, MCO-affiliated VSD researchers, scientific journals, peer reviewers for scientific journals, and people responsible for oversight of the research.

Release of Preliminary Findings When Used to Make Policy Decisions

Policy decisions or recommendations from the federal government can have a large and direct impact on the lives of Americans. The public's trust in decisions or recommendations that are based on scientific information can be affected by their trust in the scientific findings that were the basis for those decisions. The committee believes that if preliminary findings have a direct impact on a policy decision or vaccine administration guidance, the data and the findings that were the basis of that decision or guidance should be made available to the public.

> **Recommendation 4.8: The committee recommends that preliminary findings from VSD data be shared with the public whenever these findings contribute to the basis of a policy decision or are used to change guidelines on vaccine administration.**

Although "preliminary analyses" are not considered to be research data under the provisions of the Shelby Amendment, research findings may be subject to the law if they support "an agency action that has the force and effect of law" (Pub. L. No. 105-277 [1998]). The committee encourages the NIP to determine the applicability of the Shelby Amendment in situations where preliminary findings contribute to the basis of a policy decision or a change in guidelines.

Release of Preliminary Findings Superseded by Later Findings

Different considerations affect the release of preliminary findings that have already been superseded by later findings and the release of preliminary findings that represent the most recent analysis of data. In the normal scientific process, preliminary results often differ from the final results obtained through the rigorous, comprehensive analysis of a full dataset. The peer-review process is meant to ensure that final results represent the most rigorous analysis and account for confounding factors and data anomalies that were present in the preliminary results. When the peer-review process works appropriately, final results should always be considered as representing the most accurate and valid analysis of the data. However, there may be reasons to review earlier stages in the research process; for example, to determine whether and how something may have gone wrong, to allocate proper credit for scientific advances, or to simply understand scientific processes.

Because the peer-review process is designed to ensure the validity and scientific quality of the final results, preliminary findings should not be relied on as the most valid interpretations of the data. For VSD studies, the committee believes that preliminary findings superseded by later findings should not normally be released.

> **Recommendation 4.9: The committee recommends that when final results from VSD analyses or studies are released through publication or through presentation at a meeting, preliminary findings be**

shared only rarely, but that the dataset from which the final results were obtained be available to other researchers who may verify and extend the results through an audit or broader reanalysis.

Putting Preliminary Findings into Appropriate Context

Any preliminary findings that are released under the conditions specified above need to be communicated in an appropriate context. The type and degree of risk suggested by the preliminary findings will influence the public's reactions. To help the public to determine what, if any, actions to take, an indication of the public health importance of the findings should accompany their release. The public health importance of the risk and the behavior change resulting from it will be modulated by the statistical and scientific context used to communicate the risk. To portray accurately the risk conveyed by any preliminary findings from VSD data, communication about preliminary findings needs to include an assessment of the quality and integrity of the data used as the basis of the findings and possibly should include sensitivity analyses.

> **Recommendation 4.10:** The committee recommends that any preliminary findings based on VSD data that are shared with the public be put into appropriate statistical and scientific context with clear characterization of the uncertainties in the findings, of the strengths and limitations of the data, and of the possibility that new data or new analyses could change interpretations.

5

Independent Review of Vaccine Safety Datalink Activities

One of the key goals of the Vaccine Safety Datalink (VSD) data sharing program should be maintenance of public trust in the use of the VSD to draw scientific conclusions about vaccine safety. Because of the contentious nature of some of the issues surrounding the VSD and the strained relationship between the Centers for Disease Control and Prevention (CDC) and some people who have been critical of CDC's vaccine safety activities, the committee recognizes that there may be public concerns about the role of CDC in reviewing proposals to use VSD data and in setting the VSD research agenda. A perception of bias in the VSD proposal-review process and in the priorities established for the VSD research plan could jeopardize public confidence in VSD activities.

There are legitimate reasons for public concern about the independence and fairness of the review of VSD data sharing proposals and of determinations about when and how to release preliminary findings of VSD analyses. The lack of transparency of some of those processes affects the trust relationship between the National Immunization Program (NIP) and some members of the general public. To address some of those concerns, the committee believes that two independent groups should advise on different aspects of the VSD program:

1. A subcommittee of the National Vaccine Advisory Committee (NVAC) that includes representatives of a wide variety of stakeholders—such as advocacy groups, vaccine manufacturers, the Food and Drug Administration (FDA), and CDC—to review and provide advice on the VSD research plan annually.

2. An independent review committee with minimal and balanced biases and conflicts of interest to:
- Review independent external researchers' proposals to use VSD data through the data sharing program;
- Review research proposals from internal researchers and provide oversight of changes in or deviations from research protocols for internal VSD studies; and
- Provide advice on when and how preliminary findings from VSD data should be shared with the public.

The key characteristic of each of the committees is scientific independence. Independent review of the VSD research plan and of various aspects of specific VSD studies is integral to public trust in the use of the VSD to answer questions about vaccine safety.

NVAC SUBCOMMITTEE TO REVIEW AND PROVIDE ADVICE ON THE VACCINE SAFETY DATALINK RESEARCH PLAN

Every year, each VSD managed care organization (MCO) is provided an annual budget allocation. Each MCO conducts or participates in VSD studies given their available resources determined from their yearly budget. For high-priority VSD studies that require additional resources, the NIP sometimes will supplement the budget.[1] Decisions about which VSD studies should be pursued with the available resources are reached by consensus among the VSD investigators at the MCOs and the NIP.[2]

It is somewhat unclear how the priorities for the VSD research plan are set and how much input is sought from stakeholders outside the VSD steering committee. Presentations during the open sessions of the committee's meetings showed that the public also does not understand how research priorities are set.

The limitations of the VSD data sharing program and the limited ability of independent external researchers to conduct high-quality corroboration studies or studies of new hypotheses create a special need to involve the public in the priority-setting process for the VSD research plan. Only NIP-affiliated or MCO-affiliated researchers have access to VSD data for events before and after January 1, 2001, for corroboration studies and studies of new hypotheses, so independent external researchers may not be able to conduct studies that members of the public consider to have high priority. Novel hypotheses or approaches for studying previously

---

[1] Personal communication, F. DeStefano, NIP, February 10, 2005.
[2] Personal communication, F. DeStefano, NIP, February 10, 2005.

investigated hypotheses essentially cannot be pursued independently by researchers who do not wish to collaborate with other researchers or cannot find willing collaborators. In view of the limited ability of independent researchers to conduct high-quality VSD studies of new hypotheses and the limited ability of the public to provide input on which VSD studies should be pursued with federal tax dollars, there needs to be greater opportunity for input into the setting of priorities in the VSD research plan and greater transparency of the priority-setting process.

To give the full array of stakeholders an opportunity to provide input into the VSD research priority-setting process and to ensure that the process is as transparent as possible, an independent group should be used to review and provide advice on the plan. It is important that such a group represent all relevant stakeholders so that the priorities of each can be heard. Such a group should represent a broad cross-section of stakeholders and be charged with thinking strategically about VSD research priorities. The group should meet publicly and allow interested persons to observe the process and provide input through established mechanisms.

It is expected that such a group would have conflicts of interest, inasmuch as the goal would be to hear from knowledgeable persons, most of whom will be stakeholders. But the group's deliberations are also expected to occur through an open, public process. Conflicts of interest should not be avoided in a research priority-setting process meant to include all stakeholders, but the process should be transparent so that anyone can observe the deliberations that are influencing it.

The committee believes that a subcommittee of the NVAC would be the most appropriate group to review and provide advice on the VSD research plan because: (1) one of its functions is to recommend research priorities and other measures to enhance the safety and efficacy of vaccines (HHS, 2003b); (2) it includes federal officials as nonvoting ex officio members, and this allows input into the VSD research plan from other federal partners; and (3) it reports to the director of the National Vaccine Program (NVP) and is managed and supported by the NVP, which is organizationally in the Office of the Secretary of the Department of Health and Human Services. The NVAC is governed by the provisions of the Federal Advisory Committee Act (FACA). Because the NVAC is a FACA committee, the membership of the NVAC is subject to the NVAC Charter, and provisions are in place to ensure that there is public notice of meetings and that meetings are open to the public. By utilizing a subcommittee of the NVAC to review the VSD research plan annually, regular voting members of the NVAC, nonvoting ex officio members (such as CDC, FDA, and other federal agencies), and nonvoting liaison representatives (such as a representative of America's Health Insurance Plans) (HHS, 2003b) can provide input on priorities for VSD research.

The committee considered the appropriateness of having a subcommittee of the Advisory Committee on Immunization Practices (ACIP) serve this role, but it found that use of an ACIP subcommittee would not achieve the desired level of independence, because the NIP has programmatic responsibility for managing and supporting the ACIP. Use of a subcommittee of the NVAC would achieve an additional level of independence.

> **Recommendation 5.1: The committee recommends that a subcommittee of the National Vaccine Advisory Committee that includes representatives of a wide variety of stakeholders (such as advocacy groups, vaccine manufacturers, FDA, and CDC) review and provide advice to the NIP on the VSD research plan annually. The subcommittee charged with this role could be the existing Subcommittee on Safety and Communications or a subcommittee created specifically for the purpose.**

> **Recommendation 5.2: The committee recommends that the NIP propose to the National Vaccine Program that additional liaison representatives be appointed to ensure that all perspectives are heard by adequately representing advocacy groups and other members of the public at subcommittee meetings addressing the VSD research plan.**

INDEPENDENT COMMITTEE TO REVIEW VACCINE SAFETY DATALINK RESEARCH PROPOSALS AND PROVIDE ADVICE ON THE RELEASE OF PRELIMINARY FINDINGS

The committee heard about public concerns regarding the review of VSD research proposals and the procedures that independent external researchers must follow to use VSD data (Geier and Geier, 2004). Many of the specific concerns and the committee's related recommendations have been described earlier in this report. The concerns have direct implications for the release of preliminary findings.

Independence, transparency, and fairness must characterize VSD research activities if the public is to trust findings and conclusions based on VSD data. If the public questions whether the rules for access to VSD data are applied equitably to all researchers who request use of VSD data, confidence in the legitimacy of the VSD data sharing program and, ultimately, the findings from any VSD studies could be jeopardized.

Because only one group of researchers has accessed VSD data through the data sharing program, the committee could not determine whether the VSD data sharing guidelines have been applied equitably to independent external researchers. However, it has been asked to provide recommendations on any needed modifications of the data sharing program that would ensure its appropriate utilization in the future. One way to ensure fairness in utilization of the program is the creation of a committee independent of the NIP and the National Center for Health Statistics (NCHS) to review research proposals submitted by independent external researchers who request use of VSD data. Only when there is confidence that all research proposals are reviewed fairly will there be confidence in the legitimacy of all findings based on VSD data. Both the NIP and the public need a system to ensure the fair review of research proposals.

The adequacy and appropriateness of research proposals for VSD studies carried out by independent external researchers receive much scrutiny by both NCHS staff responsible for the data sharing program and the MCO Institutional Review Boards. However, it is unclear how research proposals from NIP-affiliated and MCO-affiliated researchers are evaluated. The extent to which there is oversight of NIP-affiliated and MCO-affiliated researchers' adherence to their research protocols (outlining the specification of the study population, the detailed analytic plan, sample size requirements, and study timelines) is also unclear to the public (Bernard, 2004). Lack of public confidence in adherence to detailed research protocols by researchers from the NIP or the MCOs affiliated with the VSD could jeopardize public confidence in the entire program. Especially in light of the substantial federal resources spent on the VSD program, the committee believes that the public would be served by greater transparency of VSD research activities and by assurances that all VSD research proposals are evaluated independently and that there is oversight of changes in or deviations from research protocols for internal VSD studies.

Whether, when, and how to release preliminary findings is an aspect of the VSD that needs to be characterized by independence and transparency. As the committee has outlined earlier, various conditions should govern decisions about the release of preliminary findings. The committee recognizes that not all decisions about the release of preliminary findings may fall neatly into one of these categories. The advice of an independent committee can be critical in that regard. An independent committee can evaluate the public's right to know compared with the risk of alarming the public about a risk that might not exist. The public should feel confident that the risks and benefits related to releasing such findings will always be evaluated and that an independent committee will offer advice on the most appropriate course of action.

For all those reasons, the committee believes that establishment of an independent review committee (advisory to the director of CDC) will enhance trust in the transparency and fairness of the VSD research process. It is important that an NVAC subcommittee that represents all stakeholders think strategically and provide advice on priorities for the VSD research plan, but it is also important that an operational, independent committee that is free of serious conflicts of interest review VSD research proposals and provide advice on the release of preliminary findings.

> **Recommendation 5.3: The committee recommends that an independent review committee with minimal and balanced biases and conflicts of interest be created to:**
> - **Review independent external researchers' proposals to use VSD data through the data sharing program;**
> - **Review research proposals from internal researchers and provide oversight of changes in or deviations from research protocols for internal VSD studies; and**
> - **Provide advice on when and how preliminary findings based on VSD data should be made public.**

Formation of Independent Review Committee—Criteria and Considerations

It is possible that an established committee could appropriately serve the role described here, but the committee could not identify any established committee that would be suitable. Thus, the committee concluded that an independent review committee charged with carrying out those functions should be created de novo. Whether a new committee is created or an established committee is found or reconfigured, the following criteria should guide its creation and operation:

- The committee's organization, operation, and deliberations are characterized by independence;
- Members' biases and conflicts of interest are minimal and balanced; and
- Members are chosen on the basis of scientific and technical expertise.

As long as an independent review committee meets those criteria, the committee believes that the NIP and NCHS should have flexibility in determining the structure and operating procedures of the committee. The NIP should consider having trained members of the public serve on the independent review committee if they meet the criteria of scientific and technical expertise. Matters that could be considered in the formation of such a committee include:

- Membership of the committee (number and types of members);
- Frequency of meetings;
- Staff support;

- Criteria that the committee will use to evaluate VSD research proposals;
- Process for allowing VSD program staff to provide comments on proposals;
- Which decisions or deliberations should be made public and when;
- Whether researchers or the public or both should be allowed to make presentations to the committee; and
- Types of reports or feedback provided by the committee.

The committee recognizes that the workload may be very small, at least at the beginning, and that a less weighty approach may be needed. Regardless, the three criteria listed above should still be applied.

Adherence to Protocols

When there is proper detailed documentation of research protocols, any deviations from the protocols should be clear, explicit, and adequately justified; otherwise, problems may arise. Some of the public criticisms (Bernard, 2004) of the VSD thimerosal screening study (Verstraeten et al., 2003a) were related to its alleged deviations from the original research protocol.

Good science and public accountability are enhanced when researchers adhere to original, peer-reviewed research protocols and thoroughly document and justify substantive deviations from original protocols. Transparency and public trust in the VSD would be served best by allowing an independent review committee to oversee VSD researchers' adherence to research protocols and provide advice on the best course of action if protocol deviations are not sufficiently documented and justified.

The committee encourages adherence to research protocols and documentation and justification of deviations from protocols, but it also recognizes the great benefits that may come from unstructured, unplanned research. There can be great value in informal examinations of data for unexpected signals. Such unplanned, unstructured research should not be inhibited but should be viewed as exploratory.

Appeals of Independent Review Committee Decisions

The committee recognizes that some people may dispute decisions made by the independent review committee, and an appeals process may need to be established. The entity considering the appeal should be separate from the independent review committee and should have the authority to overrule a decision of the independent review committee. The committee encourages the NIP and NCHS to establish an appeals process and specify who will be responsible for appeals decisions; the deputy director for science and public health at CDC may be an appropriate entity for this role.

Although an appeals process is needed, it is hoped that researchers and the public will trust the decisions made by the independent review committee. That will limit the number of appeals.

Concluding Remarks

The committee appreciates the opportunity to provide advice to the National Immunization Program (NIP) and the National Center for Health Statistics (NCHS) on the Vaccine Safety Datalink (VSD) data sharing program and to the NIP on the release of preliminary findings based on VSD data. The VSD database has many strengths, but it also has limitations. The value of the VSD data sharing program will be enhanced by easy access to the data so that a variety of researchers can conduct a range of studies and have their findings reviewed by peers and discussed in ways conducive to the advancement of knowledge about vaccine safety.

The VSD is a valuable resource for the nation. Efforts should be made to facilitate access to VSD data and their appropriate utilization while protecting the confidentiality of information contained therein. Ensuring the independence, transparency, and fairness of VSD research activities is important for ensuring public trust in the VSD as a tool for addressing critical vaccine safety questions.

Throughout the course of this study, the commitment of NIP and NCHS staff, of the managed care organizations participating in the VSD, of advocacy groups, and of parents to ensuring the safety of vaccines was evident to the committee. The committee believes that the debates about access to and use of VSD data have arisen from the dedication of those groups to different aspects of their common cause—ensuring vaccine safety. All the groups bring unique and important perspectives to the debate. The committee is confident that the melding of those unique perspectives will contribute to a VSD that always protects data confidentiality and is used appropriately by a wide variety of researchers to provide high-quality information on vaccine safety that will be trusted by the public.

References

Agency for Healthcare Research and Quality (AHRQ). 2004a. *CFACT Data Center (CFACT-DC)*. [Online]. Available: http://www.meps.ahrq.gov/datacenter.htm [accessed June 30, 2004].

AHRQ. 2004b. *CFACT Data Center (CFACT-DC): User Guide/Application Information*. [Online]. Available: http://www.meps.ahrq.gov/datacenter/dcuserguide.htm [accessed June 30, 2004].

AHRQ. 2004c. *Overview of the Medical Expenditure Panel Study*. [Online]. Available: http://www.meps.ahrq.gov/WhatIsMEPS/Overview.HTM [accessed June 30, 2004].

AHRQ. 2004d. *FAQs About the Data Center*. [Online]. Available: http://www.meps.ahrq.gov/FAQs/FAQ_DataCenter.HTM [accessed May, 2004].

Ball LK, Evans G, Bostrom A. 1998. Risky business: challenges in vaccine risk communication. *Pediatrics* 101(3 Pt 1):453-458.

Ball LK, Ball R, Gellin BG. 2004. Chapter 12: Developing Safe Vaccines. *New Generation Vaccines*. 3rd ed. New York: Marcel Dekker, Inc. Pp. 127-144.

Bardenheier B, Yusuf H, Schwartz B, Gust D, Barker L, Rodewald L. 2004. Are parental vaccine safety concerns associated with receipt of measles-mumps-rubella, diphtheria and tetanus toxoids with acellular pertussis, or hepatitis B vaccines by children? *Arch Pediatr Adolesc Med* 158(6):569-575.

Baylor N, Flak LA, Midthun K. 2004. Chapter 11: The Role of the Food and Drug Administration in Vaccine Testing and Licensure. *New Generation Vaccines*. 3rd ed. New York: Marcel Dekker, Inc. Pp. 117-125.

Bernard S. 2004 (October 21). *Advocacy Experience with NIP Iterative Approach to VSD Analysis & Disclosure of Preliminary Findings*. Presentation to the Committee on Review of NIP's Research Procedures and Data Sharing Program, Washington, DC.

Bernier R. 2004a (August 23). *Reflections of the NIP on the VSD Data Sharing Program*. Presentation to the Committee on Review of NIP's Research Procedures and Data Sharing Program, Washington, DC.

Bernier R. 2004b (October 21). *Charge to the IOM on Sharing Preliminary Findings from the Vaccine Safety Datalink*. Presentation to the Committee on Review of NIP's Research Procedures and Data Sharing Program, Washington, DC.

Calman KC. 2002. Communication of risk: choice, consent, and trust. *Lancet* 360(9327): 166-168.

Centers for Disease Control and Prevention (CDC). 1971. Public Health Service recommendations on smallpox vaccination. *MMWR* 20:339-345.

CDC. 1993. Pertussis Outbreaks—Massachusetts and Maryland, 1992. *MMWR* 42, 11: 197-200.

CDC. 1999a. Ten Great Public Health Achievements—United States, 1900-99. *MMWR* 48(12):241-243.

CDC. 1999b. Thimerosal in vaccines: a joint statement of the American Academy of Pediatrics and the Public Health Service. *MMWR* 48(26):563-5.

CDC. 2000. *Vaccine Safety Datalink (VSD) Project: Publications and Presentations.* [Online]. Available: http://www.cdc.gov/nip/vacsafe/vsd/references.htm [accessed June 16, 2004].

CDC. 2001. *About NIP.* [Online]. Available: http://www.cdc.gov/nip/webutil/about/default.htm [accessed November 11, 2004].

CDC. 2002. Guidelines for Data Sharing Proposals from External Researchers: Vaccine Safety Datalink (VSD) Project—Version #A. *Submitted to the Committee on Review of NIP's Research Procedures and Data Sharing Program on site visit to NIP on September 7, 2004.*

CDC. 2003a. Guidelines for Data Sharing Proposals from External Researchers: Vaccine Safety Datalink (VSD) Project—Version #B. *Submitted to the Committee on Review of NIP's Research Procedures and Data Sharing Program on site visit to NIP on September 7, 2004.*

CDC. 2003b. *CDC/ATSDR Policy on Releasing and Sharing Data.* [Online]. Available: http://www.cdc.gov/od/ads/pol-385.htm [accessed June 16, 2004].

CDC. 2003c. *NCHS Staff Manual on Confidentiality.* [Online]. Available: http://www.cdc.gov/nchs/data/misc/staffmanual2004.pdf [accessed February 11, 2005].

CDC. 2004a. Procedures and costs for use of the research data center: notice and request for action. *Federal Register* 69(222):67584-67592.

CDC. 2004b. Procedures for Use of the RDC. *Submitted via email to the Committee on Review of NIP's Research Procedures and Data Sharing Program by CDC on August 20, 2004.*

CDC. 2004c. General Description. *Submitted via email to the Committee on Review of NIP's Research Procedures and Data Sharing Program by CDC on August 20, 2004.*

CDC. 2004d. Responses to Questions Raised by the IOM Committee on the Review of NIP VSD Data Sharing Program. *Submitted via email to Committee on Review of NIP's Research Procedures and Data Sharing Program on October 4, 2004.*

CDC. 2004e. Responses to Questions Raised by the IOM Committee on the Review of NIP VSD Data Sharing Program: Appendix A. *Submitted via email to the Committee on Review of NIP's Research Procedures and Data Sharing Program by CDC on October 4, 2004.*

CDC. 2004f. Responses to Questions Raised by the IOM Committee on the Review of NIP VSD Data Sharing Program: Appendix C. *Submitted via email to the Committee on Review of NIP's Research Procedures and Data Sharing Program by CDC on October 4, 2004.*

CDC. 2004g. Procedures and costs for the use of the Research Data Center; Amendment. *Federal Register* 69(241):75316.

CDC and FDA. 2003. *Vaccine Adverse Event Reporting System (VAERS).* [Online]. Available: http://www.vaers.org/search/README.txt [accessed September 2, 2004].

CDC and FDA. 2004. *Vaccine Adverse Event Reporting System (VAERS) Data.* [Online] Available: http://www.vaers.org/info.htm [accessed September 2, 2004].

CDC and FDA. 2005. *Frequently Asked Questions About VAERS.* [Online]. Available: http://www.vaers.org/pdf/VAERS_brochure.pdf [accessed February 2005].

Census Bureau. 2004a. *CES RDC Research Proposal Guidelines.* [Online]. Available: http://148.129.75.160/ces.php/guidelines [accessed July 8, 2004].

REFERENCES

Census Bureau. 2004b. *The Research Data Center Program.* [Online]. Available at: http://148.129.75.160/ces.php/research [accessed July 8, 2004].

Chen RT. 2004. Evaluation of vaccine safety after the events of 11 September 2001: role of cohort and case-control studies. *Vaccine* 22(15-16):2047-2053.

Chen RT, Glasser JW, Rhodes PH, Davis RL, Barlow WE, Thompson RS, Mullooly JP, Black SB, Shinefield HR, Vadheim CM, Marcy SM, Ward JI, Wise RP, Wassilak SG, Hadler SC. 1997. Vaccine Safety Datalink project: a new tool for improving vaccine safety monitoring in the United States. The Vaccine Safety Datalink Team. *Pediatrics* 99(6):765-773.

California Health Interview Survey (CHIS). 2003. *CHIS Research Clearinghouse.* [Online]. Available: http://www.chis.ucla.edu/rc/ [accessed November 3, 2004].

CHIS. 2004a. *About the California Health Interview Survey.* [Online]. Available: http://www.chis.ucla.edu/about.html [accessed June 28, 2004].

CHIS. 2004b. *The Data Access Center at the UCLA Center for Health Policy Research.* [Online]. Available: http://www.chis.ucla.edu/chis_dac.html [accessed June 28, 2004].

Copeland CW, Simpson M. 2004. *The Information Quality Act: OMB's Guidance and Initial Implementation.* [Online]. Available: http://www.ombwatch.org/info/dataquality/RL32532_CRS_DQA.pdf [accessed November 18, 2004].

Council of Public Representatives (COPR) and the National Institutes of Health (NIH). 2004. *Enhancing Public Input and Transparency in the National Institutes of Health Reserach Priority-Setting Process.* [Online]. Available: http://copr.nih.gov/reports/enhancing.pdf [accessed December 29, 2004].

Cvetkovich G, Siegrist M, Murray R, Tragesser S. 2002. New information and social trust: asymmetry and perseverance of attributions about hazard managers. *Risk* 22(2): 359-367.

Davis R. 2004 (August 23). *Vaccine Safety Datalink: Overview.* Presentation to the Committee on Review of NIP's Research Procedures and Data Sharing Program, Washington, DC.

DeMets D. 2004 (October 21). *Interim Analysis of Randomized Clinical Trials.* Presentation to the Committee on Review of NIP's Research Procedures and Data Sharing Program, Washington, DC.

DeStefano F. 2004 (October 21). *VSD Studies That Utilized Iterative Analyses.* Presentation to the Committee on Review of NIP's Research Procedures and Data Sharing Program, Washington, DC.

DeStefano F, Gu D, Kramarz P, Truman BI, Iademarco MF, Mullooly JP, Jackson LA, Davis RL, Black SB, Shinefield HR, Marcy SM, Ward JI, Chen RT. 2002. Childhood vaccinations and risk of asthma. *Pediatr Infect Dis J* 21(6):498-504.

Dittmann S. 2001. Vaccine safety: risk communication—a global perspective. *Vaccine* 19(17-19):2446-2456.

Egan W. 2000. *Statement By William Egan, Ph.D., Acting Office Director, Office of Vaccine Research and Review, Center for Biologics Evaluation and Review, Food and Drug Administration, Department of Health and Human Services. Before the Committee on Government Reform: U.S. House of Representatives.* [Online]. Available: http://www.fda.gov/ola/2000/vaccines.html [accessed February 7, 2004].

Food and Drug Administration and Center for Biologics Evaluation and Research. 2002. *Vaccine Product Approval Process.* [Online]. Available: http://www.fda.gov/cber/vaccine/vacappr.htm [accessed February 3, 2005].

Fienberg S. 1994. Sharing statistical data in the biomedical and health sciences: ethical, institutional, legal, and professional dimensions. *Annual Review of Public Health* 15:1-18.

Fisher BL. 1999. *Shots in the Dark: Attempts at Eradicating Infectious Diseases Are Putting our Children at Risk.* [Online]. Available: http://www.nextcity.com/contents/summer99/16shots.html [accessed January 13, 2005].

Fisher BL. 2004a (August 23). Presentation to the Committee on Review of NIP's Research Procedures and Data Sharing Program, Washington, DC.

Fisher BL. 2004b. Statement to the Committee on Review of NIP's Research Procedures and Data Sharing Program. *Submitted to the Committee on Review of NIP's Research Procedures and Data Sharing Program on August 23, 2004.*

Government Accountability Office (GAO). 2004. Health Information: First-Year Experiences under the Federal Privacy Rule. GAO-04-965.

Geier MR, Geier DA. 2004 (August 23). *Researcher Experience with the Vaccine Safety Datalink (VSD) Data Sharing Program.* Presentation to the Committee on Review of NIP's Research Procedures and Data Sharing Program, Washington, DC.

Gellin BG, Maibach EW, Marcuse EK. 2000. Do parents understand immunizations? A national telephone survey. *Pediatrics* 106(5):1097-1102.

Gough M, Milloy S. 2000. The Case for Public Access to Federally Funded Research Data. *Cato Policy Analysis*; No. 366.

Gust DA, Strine TW, Maurice E, Smith P, Yusuf H, Wilkinson M, Battaglia M, Wright R, Schwartz B. 2004. Underimmunization among children: effects of vaccine safety concerns on immunization status. *Pediatrics* 114(1):e16-22.

Habte M. 2004 (August 23). *UCLA Center for Health Policy Research Data Access Center. UCLA Center for Health Policy Research.* Presentation to the Committee on Review of NIP's Research Procedures and Data Sharing Program, Washington, DC.

Department of Health and Human Services (HHS). 2002. *IRB Authorization Agreement.* [Online]. Available: http://www.hhs.gov/ohrp/humansubjects/assurance/iprotsup.rtf [accessed February 5, 2005].

HHS. 2003a. *Summary of the HIPAA Privacy Rule.* [Online]. Available: http://www.hhs.gov/ocr/privacysummary.pdf [accessed January 13, 2004].

HHS. 2003b. *Charter: National Vaccine Advisory Committee.* [Online]. Available: http://www.hhs.gov/nvpo/nvac/NVAC_Charter_2003.pdf [accessed February 11, 2005].

Health and Retirement Study (HRS). 2004a. *Background Information.* [Online]. Available: http://hrsonline.isr.umich.edu/intro/sho_intro.php?hfyle=uinfo [accessed June 16, 2004].

HRS. 2004b. *HRS Restricted Data: Application Processing Overview* . [Online]. Available: http://hrsonline.isr.umich.edu/rda/rdanarrative.htm [accessed July 1, 2004].

HRS. 2004c. *HRS Restricted Data: Overview.* [Online]. Available: http://hrsonline.isr.umich.edu/rda/index.html [accessed July 1, 2004].

Institute of Medicine (IOM). 1991. *Adverse Events Following Pertussis and Rubella Vaccines.* Washington, DC: National Academy Press.

Jansen VAA, Stollenwerk N, Jensen HJ, Ramsay ME, Edmunds WJ, Rhodes CJ. 2003. Measles outbreaks in a population with declining vaccine uptake. *Science* 301(August):804.

Kemp T, Pearce N, Fitzharris P, Crane J, Fergusson D, St George I, Wickens K, Beasley R. 1997. Is infant immunization a risk factor for childhood asthma or allergy? *Epidemiology* 8(6):678-680.

Mawson AR. 2001. Could bronchial asthma be an endogenous, pulmonary expression of retinoid intoxication? *Frontiers in Bioscience* 6:d973-d985.

McCall MG. 2003. *Facilitators and Barriers to Changing Health Behaviors.* [Online]. Available: http://www.medscape.com/viewarticle/466708 [accessed February 11, 2005].

McComas KA. 2004a. When even the "best-laid" plans go wrong. *European Molecular Biology Organization* 5(Special Issue):S61-S64.

McComas KA. 2004b (October 21). *Communicating Health Risks Identified Through Preliminary Analysis.* Presentation to the Committee on Review of NIP's Research Procedures and Data Sharing Program, Washington, DC.

McComas KA, Trumbo CW. 2001. Source credibility in environmental health-risk controversies: application of Meyer's credibility index. *Risk Analysis* 21(3):467-480.

McNay LA, Tavel JA, Oseekey K, McDermott CM, Mollerup D, Bebchuk JD, ESPRIT Group. 2002. Regulatory approvals in a large multinational clinical trial. *Controlled Clinical Trials* 23(1):59-66.

Mullooly J, Drew L, DeStefano F, Chen R, Okoro K, Swint E, Immanuel V, Ray P, Lewis N, Vadheim C, Lugg M. 1999. Quality of HMO vaccination databases used to monitor childhood vaccine safety. Vaccine Safety DataLink Team. *Am J Epidemiol* 149(2):186-194.

National Academy of Sciences (NAS), National Academy of Engineering (NAE), Institute of Medicine (IOM). 1996. *On Being a Scientist: Responsible Conduct in Research.* Washington, DC: National Academy Press.

National Institutes of Health (NIH). 2004a. *NIH Data Sharing Policy.* [Online]. Available: http://grants.nih.gov/grants/policy/data_sharing/ [accessed June 16, 2004].

NIH. 2004b. *Notice: Enhanced Public Access to NIH Research Information.* [Online]. Available: http://grants1.nih.gov/grants/guide/notice-files/NOT-OD-04-064.html [accessed January 14, 2004].

NIH. 2005a. *Director's Council on Public Representatives (COPR).* [Online]. Available: http://copr.nih.gov [accessed January 11, 2005].

NIH. 2005b. *NIH Calls on Scientists to Speed Public Release of Research Publications.* [Online]. Available: http://www.nih.gov/news/pr/feb2005/od-03.htm [accessed February 4, 2005].

National Research Council (NRC) and Committee on National Statistics. 1985. *Sharing Research Data.* Washington, DC: National Academy Press.

National Vaccine Information Center (NVIC). 2004. *National Vaccine Information Center Says IOM Played Politics in Report on Autism and Vaccines.* [Online]. Available: http://www.nvic.org/PressReleases/pr51804iom.htm [accessed January 13, 2005].

Offit PA, Coffin SE. 2003. Communicating science to the public: MMR vaccine and autism. *Vaccine* 22(1):1-6.

Office of Management and Budget (OMB). 1999. OMB Circular A-110, uniform administrative requirements for grants and agreements with institutions of higher education, hospitals, and other non-profit organizations. *Federal Register* 64(195):54926-54930.

Phillips K. 2002. *Public Access to Research Data.* [Online]. Available: http://depts.washington.edu/ventures/About_Us/Presentations/Data_Rights/Public_Access.ppt [accessed February 11, 2005].

Pless R, Casey C, Chen R, and Vaccine Safety and Development Activity. 2004. *Clinical Immunization Safety Assessment Centers: Improving the Evaluation, Management and Understanding of Adverse Events Possibly Related to Immunizations.* [Online]. Available: http://www.cdc.gov/nip/vacsafe/cisa/intro-cisa.pdf [accessed February 4, 2005].

Poortinga W, Pidgeon NF. 2004. Trust, the asymmetry principle, and the role of prior beliefs. *Risk* 24(6):1475-1486.

SafeMinds. 2003. Analysis and critque of the CDC's handling of the thimerosal exposure assessment based on Vaccine Safety Datalink (VSD) information. *Submitted by S. Bernard on Behalf of SAFEMINDS on 1/18/04 to the Immunization Safety Review Committee*: 1-46.

SafeMinds. 2004a. *A Brief Analysis of Recent Efforts in Medical Mercury Induced Neurological and Autism Spectrum Disorders.* [Online]. Available: http://www.safeminds.org/pressroom/press_releases/08Sep2004_A_Brief_Analysis.html#_Toc82334450 [accessed January 13, 2005].

SafeMinds. 2004b. *SafeMinds Outraged That IOM Report Fails American Public.* [Online]. Available: http://www.safeminds.org/pressroom/press_releases/040518-PR10-BadIOMReport.pdf [accessed January 13, 2005].

Siegrist M, Cvetkovich G. 2001. Better negative than positive? Evidence of a bias for negative information about possible health dangers. *Risk* 21(1):199-206.

Simpsonwood Transcript. 2000. Scientific Review of Vaccine Safety Datalink Information, June 7-8, 2000. Simpsonwood Retreat Center, Norcross, GA.

Slovic P. 1987. Perception of risk. *Science* 236(4799):280-285.

Slovic P. 1993. Perceived risk, trust and democracy. *Risk Analysis* 13:675-682.

Verstraeten T. 2001. Presentation to Immunization Safety Review Committee. *Vaccine Safety Datalink (VSD) Screening Study and Follow-Up Analysis with Harvard Pilgrim Data*, Washington, DC.

Verstraeten T, Davis RL, DeStefano F, Lieu TA, Rhodes PH, Black SB, Shinefield H, Chen RT, Vaccine Safety Datalink Team. 2003a. Safety of thimerosal-containing vaccines: a two-phased study of computerized health maintenance organization databases. *Pediatrics* 112(5):1039-1048.

Verstraeten T, DeStefano F, Chen RT, Miller E . 2003b. Vaccine safety surveillance using large linked databases: opportunities, hazards and proposed guidelines. *Expert Rev Vaccines* 2(1):21-29.

Weijer C. 2004 (October 21). *When to release preliminary findings: Ethical considerations*. Presentation to the Committee on Review of NIP's Research Procedures and Data Sharing Program, Washington, DC.

Wharton M. 2004 (August 23). *The Vaccine Safety Datalink (VSD) Data Sharing Program*. Presentation to the Committee on Review of NIP's Research Procedures and Data Sharing Program, Washington, DC.

World Health Organization (WHO). 2005. *Vaccine Safety Websites Meeting Essential and Important Good Information Practices Criteria*. [Online]. Available: http://www.who.int/immunization_safety/safety_quality/approved_vaccine_safety_websites/en/ [accessed January 13, 2005].

Appendix A

Committee Biographies

**COMMITTEE ON THE REVIEW OF THE
NATIONAL IMMUNIZATION PROGRAM'S RESEARCH
PROCEDURES AND DATA SHARING PROGRAM**

John C. Bailar III *(Committee Chair)*, M.D, Ph.D., is Professor Emeritus in the Department of Health Studies at the University of Chicago. He is a retired commissioned officer of the U.S. Public Health Service, and worked for the National Cancer Institute for 22 years. He has also held academic appointments at Harvard University and McGill University. He was editor-in-chief of the *Journal of the National Cancer Institute* for six years, and was a statistical consultant and member of the editorial board for the *New England Journal of Medicine*. Dr. Bailar is a member of the International Statistical Institute. He has been the chair of several Institute of Medicine (IOM) and National Research Council (NRC) committees. Dr. Bailar's research interests include interpreting statistical evidence in medicine, with special emphasis on cancer. He received his M.D. from Yale University and his Ph.D. in statistics from American University. Dr. Bailar is a member of the IOM.

Garnet L. Anderson, Ph.D., is the Co-Principal Investigator of the Women's Health Initiative Clinical Coordinating Center. She is also a member of the Public Health Sciences Division, the associate program head of the Gynecologic Cancer Program at the Fred Hutchinson Cancer Research Center, and affiliate associate professor in the Department of

Biostatistics at the University of Washington. Dr. Anderson has been affiliated with the Women's Health Initiative in numerous capacities since 1993. She has served as associate editor of Controlled Clinical Trials and Clinical Journal of Women's Health. Dr. Anderson's research interests include the design, analysis, and conduct of clinical trials, data monitoring, survival analysis, women's health, and ovarian cancer. She received her Ph.D. in biostatistics from the University of Washington.

Stephen E. Fienberg, Ph.D., is Maurice Falk University Professor of Statistics and Social Science at Carnegie Mellon University. He previously was Professor of Statistics and Law at York University. Dr. Fienberg is a fellow of the American Association for the Advancement of Science, the American Academy of Political and Social Science, the American Statistical Association, the Institute of Mathematical Statistics, and the Royal Statistical Society. He has chaired and served on several IOM and NRC committees, including serving as chair of the CNSTAT Subcommittee on Data Sharing that produced the NRC report "Sharing Research Data" in 1985. Dr. Fienberg's research interests include the development of statistical methodology, especially for problems involving categorical variables; disclosure limitation for statistical databases; statistical methods for large-scale sample surveys, such as those carried out by the federal government; the study of nonsampling errors; and formal parallels in the design and analysis of sample surveys and randomized experiments. He received his Ph.D. in statistics from Harvard University. Dr. Fienberg is a member of the National Academy of Sciences and a fellow of the Royal Society of Canada.

Debra R. Lappin, J.D., is Senior Advisor to B&D Sagamore, a Washington, DC-based public policy firm. Ms. Lappin serves as a consultant to industry, academic research institutions, nonprofit entities, and government on the structure and execution of collaborative cross-sector partnerships, on the development and implementation of public health initiatives, and on mechanisms for public engagement in science and enhancing public trust as an institutional asset. From 1996 to 1998, Ms. Lappin was the Chair of the Arthritis Foundation. She was a charter member of the National Institutes of Health (NIH) Director's Council of Public Representatives from 1999 to 2003, and chaired its working group on Human Research Protections. Ms. Lappin lectures as an adjunct faculty member in the Department of Medicine, University of Colorado Health Sciences Center, chairs the Ethics Committee at National Jewish Medical and Research Center in Denver, and speaks often on the subject of the new partnership between the public and the scientific enterprise. Ms. Lappin has served on the IOM Committee on the Organizational Structure of the

National Institutes of Health and the Committee on Changing Health Care Systems and Rheumatic Disease. Ms. Lappin received her J.D. from the University of Denver.

Myron M. Levine, M.D., D.T.P.H., is Professor and Director of the Center for Vaccine Development at the University of Maryland School of Medicine. During his 34 years at the University, he has fostered the discipline of vaccinology, focusing on basic research on the pathogenesis of bacterial enteric infections and on the construction of vaccine candidates; clinical research to assess the safety and immunogenicity of candidate vaccines in adult and pediatric populations; and epidemiological field research. Dr. Levine has served on the IOM Committee on the Review of the USDA *E. coli* 0157:H7 Farm-to-Table Process Risk Assessment, the Steering Committee for the Study on the U.S. Capacity to Address Tropical Disease Problems, and is a member of the Board of the Medical Follow-Up Agency. He received his M.D. from the Medical College of Virginia and completed a pediatric residency and pediatric infectious disease fellowship at the Albert Einstein College of Medicine. Dr. Levine received his D.T.P.H. from the London School of Hygiene and Tropical Medicine. Dr. Levine is a member of the IOM.

Anna C. Mastroianni, J.D., M.P.H., is an Assistant Professor at the School of Law and at the Institute for Public Health Genetics at the University of Washington. Previously, Professor Mastroianni was a practicing health care attorney, Associate Director of the White House Advisory Committee on Human Radiation Experiments, and a study director for the IOM Committee to Study the Legal and Ethical Issues Relating to the Inclusion of Women in Clinical Studies. Her research and teaching focus on health law and bioethics, with specific interests in the legal, ethical, and policy issues related to the responsible conduct of research, human subjects research, public health, the use of genetic technologies, and women's health. Professor Mastroianni is a fellow of the American Association for the Advancement of Science. She has served on the NRC Committee on Institutional Review Boards, Surveys, and Social Science Research. Professor Mastroianni received her J.D. from the University of Pennsylvania Law School and her M.P.H. from the University of Washington School of Public Health and Community Medicine. She is the author and coauthor of numerous publications on law, ethics, and public health policy.

Colin L. Soskolne, Ph.D., is Professor of Epidemiology in the Department of Public Health Sciences at the University of Alberta, where he has been based since 1985. Following graduate studies, he was Director of the Epidemiology Research Unit of the Ontario Cancer Treatment and Research Foundation at the University of Toronto. In 1999, he completed a sabbatical year as Visiting Scientist with the World Health Organization's European Centre for Environment and Health in Rome, Italy. Dr. Soskolne spearheaded efforts to bring the question of professional ethics into focus for epidemiologists world wide. He was the first to call for ethics guidelines for epidemiologists in his paper in the *Journal of Public Health Policy* in 1985, and has jointly published ethics guidelines for environmental epidemiologists. He is a fellow and an elected officer in the American College of Epidemiology. Dr. Soskolne's research interests include professional ethics in epidemiology, the health effects of occupational exposure to acid mists, and ecological disintegrity in relation to human health and well-being. Dr. Soskolne received his Ph.D. in epidemiology from the University of Pennsylvania. He won the Society for Epidemiologic Research annual student prize in 1983 for his Ph.D. thesis.

Elaine Vaughan, Ph.D., is Associate Professor of Psychology in the Department of Psychology and Social Behavior at the University of California, Irvine. She currently is involved in a longitudinal field experiment assessing the effects of participatory decision strategies for high-priority waste sites on social conflict and community response to risk. Her research interests include public understanding and use of scientific risk information, the interplay among cultural values/beliefs and emotional or cognitive response to risk, socioeconomic context of exposure and response to environmental risk, risk communication, risk perceptions of culturally diverse populations, and measurement and statistical issues that arise when studying psychosocial phenomena across diverse populations. Recently, she has published articles on risk communication and individual and community response to bioterrorism. Dr. Vaughan has served on the NRC Panel on Public Participation in Environmental Assessment and Decision Making, the IOM Committee on Strategies to Protect the Health of Deployed U.S. Forces, and the NRC Committee on Risk Characterization. Dr. Vaughan received her Ph.D. in social psychology from Stanford University.

Appendix B

Glossary

Please Note: The definitions used here represent their meaning for use in this report and may not have the same meaning when used in other contexts.

Audit: The recalculation of statistics included in a previous study report using the same final analytic dataset.

Broader Reanalysis: The examination of variables or possibly individuals omitted from the final dataset, but would not usually involve the entire source dataset.

Confidentiality: The prevention of the unauthorized disclosure of personal information.

Corroboration Study: A test of the same hypothesis using a new design or study population.

Data Enclave: A controlled, secure environment in which eligible researchers can perform analyses using data resources with restrictions on the level of identifiable entities that may be removed from the enclave.

Data Sharing Program: A program to allow researchers access to data collected by another entity.

External Researcher: A researcher who is not affiliated with an institution that is the data owner or the data steward.

Findings: The results of an investigation that are deemed final given the nature and extent of the work done.

Institutional Review Board: A committee formally established by a research institution to ensure that the rights and welfare of human subjects are protected.

Internal Researcher: A researcher who is affiliated with an institution that is the data owner or the data steward.

Investigation of a New Hypothesis: A new study of a previously untested hypothesis.

Managed Care Organization (MCO): (also referred to as **Health Maintenance Organization (HMO)**) A health care organization that, in return for prospective per capita (capitation) payments, integrates financing, care delivery, resource allocation, and quality assurance. A prepaid delivery system in which the organization (and usually its primary care physicians) assumes financial risk for the care provided to enrolled members. The organization is legally committed to provide care to its enrollees, and members must obtain care from within the system if it is to be reimbursed.

Preliminary Data: The underlying elements of information of a study or investigation which are still incomplete or subject to change.

Preliminary Findings: Initial results obtained from investigations or studies often expressed in summary statements or summary-like form such as tables or graphs. These results are incomplete and subject to change prior to peer-reviewed publication.

Research: Systematic investigation, including research development, testing, and evaluation, designed to develop or contribute to generalizable knowledge.

Surveillance: Regular, ongoing collection and analysis of data to monitor the occurrence of health problems.

Technical Feasibility: The requested data are available in the database, there are enough individuals in the database with the exposures and outcomes of interest to study the proposed hypothesis, and the proposed statistical tests are possible with the available data.

Appendix C

Acronyms

ACIP – Advisory Committee on Immunization Practices
ADHD – Attention Deficit Hyperactivity Disorder
AHRQ – Agency for Healthcare Research and Quality

BLA – Biologics License Application

CBER – Center for Biologics Evaluation and Research
CDC – Centers for Disease Control and Prevention
CES – Center for Economic Studies
CFACT-DC – Center for Financing, Access, and Cost Trends Data Center
CFR – Code of Federal Regulations
CHIS – California Health Interview Survey
CIPSEA – Confidential Information Protection and Statistical Efficiency Act of 2002
CISA – Clinical Immunization Safety Assessment
CNSTAT – Committee on National Statistics
COPR – Council of Public Representatives

DAC – Data Access Center
DCC – Data Confidentiality Committee
DCC-WG – Data Confidentiality Committee Working Group

FDA – Food and Drug Administration
FOIA – Freedom of Information Act

GPRD – General Practice Research Database
GVAC – Global Vaccine Advisory Committee

HHS – Department of Health and Human Services
HIPAA – Health Insurance Portability and Accountability Act
HRS – Health and Retirement Study

ICAAC– Interscience Conference on Antimicrobial Agents and Chemotherapy
IND – Investigational New Drug
IOM – Institute of Medicine
IQA – Information Quality Act
IRB – Institutional Review Board

MCO – Managed Care Organization
MEPS – Medical Expenditure Panel Survey
MiCDA – Michigan Center on the Demography of Aging

NCHS – National Center for Health Statistics
NIH – National Institutes of Health
NIP – National Immunization Program
NRC – National Research Council
NVAC – National Vaccine Advisory Committee

OMB – Office of Management and Budget

RDC – Research Data Center

VAERS – Vaccine Adverse Event Reporting System
VRBPAC – Vaccines and Related Biological Products Advisory Committee
VSD – Vaccine Safety Datalink

WHO – World Health Organization

Appendix D

Meeting One—Agenda

The National Academies
Institute of Medicine

Committee on Review of NIP's Research Procedures and
Data Sharing Program
Meeting One

AGENDA

Speakers and Times Subject to Change

Monday, August 23, 2004
10:30 a.m. – 5:45 p.m.

Meeting Location: Keck Center of the National Academies
Room 100
500 Fifth Street, NW
Washington, DC 20001

10:00 – 10:30 a.m.   Registration and Coffee

10:30 – 10:45 a.m.	Welcome, Introductions, and Opening Statement *John Bailar, MD, PhD* Committee Chair
10:45 – 10:55 a.m.	Description of the Vaccine Safety Datalink (VSD) *Robert Davis, MD, MPH* Visiting Scientist Office of Genomics and Disease Prevention Centers for Disease Control and Prevention
10:55 – 11:15 a.m.	Background on the NCHS Research Data Center (RDC) *Jennifer Madans, PhD* Associate Director for Science National Center for Health Statistics Centers for Disease Control and Prevention
11:15 – 11:40 a.m.	Description of the VSD Data Sharing Program *Melinda Wharton, MD, MPH* Acting Deputy Director National Immunization Program Centers for Disease Control and Prevention
11:40 – 11:45 a.m.	Future Plans for the VSD Data Sharing Program *Jennifer Madans, PhD*
11:45 a.m. – 12:05 p.m.	Questions from the Committee
12:05 – 12:15 p.m.	Charge to the Committee *Roger Bernier, PhD, MPH* Senior Advisor For Scientific Strategy and Innovation National Immunization Program Centers for Disease Control and Prevention
12:15 – 12:30 p.m.	Questions from the Committee
12:30 – 1:15 p.m.	Lunch (Cafeteria on 3rd Floor)

APPENDIX D 121

1:15 – 1:45 p.m.	Researchers' Experience with the VSD Data Sharing Program *Mark R. Geier, MD, PhD* President The Genetic Centers of America *David Geier* President MedCon
1:45 – 2:15 p.m.	Questions from the Committee
2:15 – 2:25 p.m.	RDC Monitor's Experience with the VSD Data Sharing Program *Peter Shabe, MS* Director of Data Management and Statistics TrialTech
2:25 – 2:40 p.m.	NIP's Experience with the VSD Data Sharing Program *Roger Bernier, PhD, MPH*
2:40 – 3:00 p.m.	Questions from the Committee
3:00 – 3:10 p.m.	Break
3:10 – 3:30 p.m.	Perspective and Experience of a Managed Care Organization Involved in the VSD Data Sharing Program *Richard Platt, MD, MSc* Professor and Chair Department of Ambulatory Care and Prevention Harvard Medical School Harvard Pilgrim Health Care
3:30 – 3:45 p.m.	Questions from the Committee
3:45 – 4:05 p.m.	Access to California Health Interview Survey Data through the UCLA Data Access Center *Lee Habte, MA* Data Access Center Manager UCLA Center for Health Policy Research

4:05 – 4:20 p.m.	Questions from the Committee
4:20 – 4:40 p.m.	Perspective of a Consumer Group on Access to VSD Data *Barbara Loe Fisher* President National Vaccine Information Center
4:40 – 4:55 p.m.	Questions from the Committee
4:55 – 5:40 p.m.	Public Comment *(A sign-up sheet will be available at the registration table)*
5:40 – 5:45 p.m.	Closing Remarks *John Bailar, MD, PhD* Committee Chair

Appendix E

Meeting Two—Agenda

The National Academies
Institute of Medicine

Committee on Review of NIP's Research Procedures and
Data Sharing Program
Meeting Two

AGENDA

Speakers and Times Subject to Change

Thursday, October 21, 2004
9:00 a.m. – 5:30 p.m.

Meeting Location:	Keck Center of the National Academies Room 100 500 Fifth Street, NW Washington, DC 20001
8:30 – 9:00 a.m.	Registration and Coffee

9:00 – 9:15 a.m.	Welcome, Introductions, and Opening Statement *John Bailar, MD, PhD* Committee Chair
9:15 – 9:35 a.m.	Charge to the Committee—Second Component of Charge *Roger Bernier, PhD, MPH* Senior Advisor for Scientific Strategy and Innovation National Immunization Program Centers for Disease Control and Prevention
9:35 – 9:50 a.m.	Questions from the Committee
9:50 – 10:10 a.m.	A Peer-Reviewed Journal's Perspective on the Release of Preliminary Findings *Harold Sox, MD* Editor Annals of Internal Medicine American College of Physicians of Internal Medicine
10:10 – 10:25 a.m.	Questions from the Committee
10:25 – 10:40 a.m.	Break
10:40 – 11:00 a.m.	When to Release Preliminary Findings: Ethical Considerations *Charles Weijer, MD, PhD, FRCPC* CIHR Investigator Associate Professor of Bioethics, Medicine, and Surgery Adjunct Professor of Philosophy Department of Bioethics Dalhousie Medical School
11:00 – 11:15 a.m.	Questions from the Committee

11:15 – 11:35 a.m.	Communicating Health Risks Identified Through Preliminary Analyses *Katherine McComas, PhD* Assistant Professor Department of Communication Cornell University
11:35 – 11:50 a.m.	Questions from the Committee
11:50 – 12:10 p.m.	When to Release Preliminary Findings: Post-Market Surveillance of Medical Devices *Susan Gardner, PhD* Director, Office of Surveillance Biometrics Center for Devices and Radiological Health Food and Drug Administration
12:10 – 12:25 p.m.	Questions from the Committee
12:25 – 1:30 p.m.	Lunch (Cafeteria on 3rd Floor; List of nearby restaurants in folder)
1:30 – 2:00 p.m.	VSD Studies that Utilized Iterative Analyses *Frank DeStefano, MD, MPH* Medical Epidemiologist National Immunization Program Centers for Disease Control and Prevention
2:00 – 2:15 p.m.	Questions from the Committee
2:15 – 2:35 p.m.	Statistical Methods and Issues Relevant to Iterative Analyses *David DeMets, PhD* Professor and Chair Department of Biostatistics and Medical Informatics University of Wisconsin-Madison
2:35 – 2:50 p.m.	Questions from the Committee

2:50 – 3:10 p.m.	Use of Preliminary Findings for Policy Decisions: The Rotavirus Vaccine Experience *Melinda Wharton, MD, MPH* Acting Deputy Director National Immunization Program Centers for Disease Control and Prevention
3:10 – 3:25 p.m.	Questions from the Committee
3:25 – 3:40 p.m.	Break
3:40 – 4:00 p.m.	Advocacy Group Perspective on Criteria for Releasing Preliminary Findings *Sallie Bernard* Executive Director and Co-Founder SafeMinds
4:00 – 4:15 p.m.	Questions from the Committee
4:15 – 4:35 p.m.	Pediatricians' Perspective on Preliminary Findings as Evidence for Decision-Making *Julia McMillan, MD* Professor of Pediatrics Vice Chair for Pediatric Education Johns Hopkins University School of Medicine
4:35 – 4:50 p.m.	Questions from the Committee
4:50 – 5:20 p.m.	Public Comment *(A sign-up sheet will be available at the registration table)*
5:20 – 5:30 p.m.	Closing Remarks *John Bailar, MD, PhD* Committee Chair

Appendix F

Summary of Public Submissions

The committee has received numerous public submissions and comments via e-mail, fax, and mail since the announcement of its first meeting in August 2004. The submissions were reviewed by the committee to inform its recommendations for this report.

All information reviewed by the committee and cited in this report are available—in the form in which they were reviewed—through the public-access files of the National Academies. Information about this process and access to these documents can be obtained at 202-334-3543 or www.national-academies.org/publicaccess.

Below is a list as of February 11, 2005, of the public submissions received, divided into three categories.

1) Personal Statements

The committee received many statements from the public that described their views on the Vaccine Safety Datalink data sharing program and the release of preliminary findings from the VSD. The committee also received personal statements about vaccines and autism in general:

- Barile, D. Data Base. September 1, 2004.
- Bono, L. and Bono, S. (National Autism Association). Submitted Testimony. October 21, 2004.
- Brasher, A. Thimerosal. August 31, 2004.
- Brown, W. Vaccine Safety Datalink. September 2, 2004.
- Buckley, P. Vaccine Data Base. September 1, 2004.

- Conrick, T. To IOM Committee on Review of NIP's Research Procedures and Data Sharing Program. September 3, 2004.
- Cook, B, and Cook, L. Vaccine Safety Datalink. September 2, 2004.
- Dakdouk, D. Vaccine Safety Datalink. September 1, 2004.
- Dannemann, E. (Director, National Caalition of Organized Women). Letter submitted to the Committee on Review of NIP's Research Procedures and Data Sharing Program. August 23, 2004.
- Dannemann, E. (Director, National Caalition of Organized Women). Letter with multiple attachments: Comments on Data Sharing. August 27, 2004.
- Dannemann, E. (Director, National Caalition of Organized Women) Statement for IOM Hearing 8/23/04 on Vaccine Safety Datalink Access to Public, by A. Gore. August 27, 2004.
- Davidson, L. To IOM Committee on Review of NIP's Research Procedures and Data Sharing Program. September 16, 2004.
- Dease, B. IOM Meeting. September 1, 2004.
- Fisher, B.L. (National Vaccine Information Center). Statement to the Committee on Review of NIP's Research Procedures and Data Sharing Program. August 23, 2004.
- Greenwood, J. Autism. December 16, 2004.
- Greenwood, J. VSD. August 31, 2004.
- Hale, E. Sharing info. September 2, 2004.
- Hanus, L. Letter to the Committee on Review of NIP's Research Procedures and Data Sharing Program. August 23, 2004.
- Kalika, D. and Kalika, E. Vaccine Safety Datalink. August 31, 2004.
- Kanji, S. VSD Data Access. August 31, 2004.
- King, P. A Poisoned Child's Cry. August 23, 2004.
- Krumenacker, J. Review of NIP's Research Procedures and Data Sharing Program met last week to discuss future handling of the Vaccine Safety Datalink. August 31, 2004.
- Lathrop, H. Regarding data sharing. August 20, 2004.
- Maniotis, R. Letter to Committee on Review of NIP's Research Procedures and Data Sharing Program. August 23, 2004.
- McCandless, J. Letter to the Committee on Review of NIP's Research Procedures and Data Sharing Program. August 19, 2004.
- McCandless, J. A physician shares a letter from a parent to the IOM. August 29, 2004.
- McCandless, J. McC to IOM. August 31, 2004.
- McDonald, M.E. Comments—Access to VSD September 1, 2004.
- Meleck, M. VSD. September 1, 2004.
- Mumper, E. Letter to the Committee on Review of NIP's Research Procedures and Data Sharing Program. August 23, 2004.

APPENDIX F   129

- National Vaccine Information Center (NVIC), submitted by B.L. Fischer. Petition. October 21, 2004.
- Phipps, S. IOM Input. August 31, 2004.
- Piselli, J. and Piselli, P. Autism. September 6, 2004.
- Piselli, J. and Piselli, P. VSD Access. September 12, 2004.
- Ranieri, S. Comments on data sharing on vaccines. September 24, 2004.
- Rankin, D. We had a perfectly normal grandson. August 31, 2004.
- Thompson, J. Please release the VSD information. September 2, 2004.
- vanDoorn, C. Access to VSD. September 2, 2004.
- VanHaaften, J. Comments on data sharing on vaccines. August 19, 2004.
- Vernetti, S. VSD Comments. August 31, 2004.
- Weed, L. VSD. September 14, 2004.
- Weinmaster, L. VSD. September 1, 2004.

2) Questions to Consider

Several people e-mailed questions to the committee for them to consider while reviewing its charge, and making its recommendations. They included:

- Bernard, S.
- Enayati, A.
- Krakow, R.
- Peterson, M.
- Wax, M.

3) Documents for Review

The committee received many published and unpublished documents:

- ACIP Charter. *(Submitted by M. Wharton, October 2004)*
- Amendment of Solicitation/Modification of Contract between NIP and HMOs involved in the VSD Data Sharing Program dated February 2003 – October 2004 *(Submitted by NIP, 2004)*
- Award/Contract 200-2002-00732, Effective Date 09/20/2002 *(Submitted by NIP, 2004)*
- Clarification of the draft VSD data sharing guidelines *(Submitted by J. Madans and K. Harris at NIP, February 2005)*
- Clarification of your presentation to the IOM on October 21, 2004:

Responses to your questions *(Submitted by F. DeStefano via P. Harvey on February 10, 2005)*
- Cochlear Implant Recipients may be at Greater Risk for Meningitis by FDA, 2002. *(Submitted by S. Gardner on October 21, 2004)*
- Correspondence between W. Broom and M. Geier dated November 2002–September 2004. *(Submitted by NIP, 2004)*
- Confidentiality Security Statement, Vaccine Safety Datalink Project (VSD). *(Submitted by NIP, October 2004)*
- Current Legislative Authorities Pamphlet, 2000. *(Submitted by the National Center for Health Statistics (NCHS) on committee site visit to NCHS on September 22, 2004)*
- Evidence of Harm—*Book Cover only* by Kirby D. *(Submitted by L. and S. Bono, October 2004)*
- FDA Public Health Web Notification: Information for Physicians on Sub-acute Thromboses (SAT) and Hypersensitivity Reactions with Use of the Cordis CYPHER™ Coronary Stent by FDA, 2003. *(Submitted by S. Gardner on October 21, 2004)*
- FDA Public Health Web Notification: Risk of Bacterial Meningitis in Children with Cochlear Implants by FDA, 2003. *(Submitted by S. Gardner on October 21, 2004)*
- FDA Public Health Web Notification: Updated Information for Physicians on Sub-acute Thromboses (SAT) and Hypersensitivity Reactions with Use of the Cordis CYPHER™ Sirolimus-eluting Coronary Stent by FDA, 2003. *(Submitted by S. Gardner on October 21, 2004)*
- Genetic Disclosure Project. *(Submitted by M. Gordon on October 15, 2004)*
- Guidelines for Data Sharing Proposals from External Researchers: Vaccine Safety Datalink (VSD) Project—Version #A, 2002. *(Submitted by NIP on committee site visit to NIP on September 7, 2004)*
- Guidelines for Data Sharing Proposals from External Researchers: Vaccine Safety Datalink (VSD) Project—Version #B, 2003. *(Submitted by NIP on committee site visit to NIP on September 7, 2004)*
- It just won't go away. *E-mail to Davis R, DeStefano from Verstraeten T, 1999. (Submitted by M. Geier on October 21, 2004)*
- J & J stent linked to more than 60 deaths by Kerber R, (Boston Globe Staff), 2003. *(Submitted by S. Gardner on October 21, 2004)*
- Letter to John Bailar and Committee on Review of NIP's Research Procedures and Data Sharing Program by D. Weldon. *(Submitted by Congressman Dave Weldon on September 13, 2004)*
- NCHS Research Data Center Pamphlet, 2001. *(Submitted by NCHS on committee site visit to NIP on September 22, 2004)*
- NCHS Staff manual on Confidentiality, 2004. *(Submitted by NCHS on committee site visit to NIP on September 7, 2004)*

- Press Packet (Folder) by SafeMinds, National Autism Association, Moms Against Mercury, Nomercury.org, BC&A International, Unlocking Autism, Coalition for Mercury Free Drugs, Autism Autoimmunity Project. *(Joint Statement: Submitted to the Committee on Review of NIP's Research Procedures and Data Sharing Program on August 23, 2004)*
- Professional paper by Russell Blaylock, MD. *(Submitted by L.J. O'Brien, September 1, 2004)*
- Responses to questions raised by the IOM Committee on the Review of NIP VSD Data Sharing Program, with attachments A-E. *(Submitted by NIP on October 4, 2004)*
- Summary Statistics—Thimerosal Study: Attachment #1 by D. Weldon. *(Submitted by Congressman Dave Weldon on September 17, 2004)*
- TrialTech Visit as Technical Monitor to the NCHS RDC, by Adelman T, Shabe P, 2004. *(Submitted by National Immunization Program [NIP], November 2004)*
- Vaccine Safety Datalink Project, Confidentiality Assurance Statement. *(Submitted by NIP on October 6, 2004)*
- VSD Contract with attachment A-J. *(Submitted by NIP on October 6, 2004)*
- Safety of Thimerosal-Containing Vaccines: A Two-Phased Study of Computerized Health Maintenance Organization Databases by Verstraeton et al., 2003. *(Submitted by Congressman Dave Weldon on September 17, 2004)*
- Judgement Under Uncertainty: Suspending the Use of Rotavirus Vaccine by M. Wharton (CDC), 2000. *(Submitted by M. Wharton on October 21, 2004)*
- Mothering Magazine. No. 125. *(Submitted by L. Sykes on August 23, 2004)*
- Guidelines for Archival Datasets and Documentation from Completed Vaccines Safety Datalink (VSD) Studies; Draft 4.0. *(Submitted by NIP November 2004)*
- General Description. *(Submitted by J. Madans on August 20, 2004)*
- Procedures for Use of the RDC. *(Submitted by J. Madans on August 20, 2004)*
- Progressive Convergence. Do Not Vaccinate Your Child Without Due Diligence. Find Out About Mercury in Their Vaccinations. *(Submitted by Progressive Convergence on August 24, 2004)*
- Thimerosal paper in Frank DeStefano's presentation in October. *(Submitted by P. Harvey on December 9, 2004)*
- Letter to F. Pavley by J. McCandless. *(Submitted by J. McCandless on August 13, 2004)*

Appendix G

Notice and Request for Comment on *Procedures and Costs for Use of the Research Data Center*

APPENDIX G

2000, the Department of Health and Human Services (HHS) has been given the responsibility and resources for conducting analytic epidemiologic investigations of residents of communities in the vicinity of DOE facilities, workers at DOE facilities, and other persons potentially exposed to radiation or to potential hazards from non-nuclear energy production and use. HHS has delegated program responsibility to CDC. Community involvement is a critical part of ATSDR's and CDC's energy-related research and activities and input from members of the ORRHES is part of these efforts.

Purpose: The purpose of this meeting is to address issues that are unique to community involvement with the ORRHES, and agency updates.

Matters to be Discussed: Agenda items will include a brief discussion on the ATSDR project management plan and the schedule of Public Health Assessments to be released in FY2005–2006, and updates and recommendations from the Exposure Evaluation, Community Concerns and Communications, and the Health Outcome Data Workgroups, and agency updates.

Agenda items are subject to change as priorities dictate.

Due to programmatic issues that had to be resolved, the **Federal Register** notice is being published less than fifteen days before the date of the meeting.

Contact Persons for More Information: Marilyn Horton, Designated Federal Official and Committee Management Specialist, Division of Health Assessment and Consultation, ATSDR, 1600 Clifton Road, NE., M/S E–32 Atlanta, Georgia 30333, telephone 1–888–42–ATSDR (28737), fax (404) 498–1744.

The Director, Management Analysis and Services Office, has been delegated the authority to sign **Federal Register** notices pertaining to announcements of meetings and other committee management activities, for both CDC and ATDSR.

Dated: November 10, 2004.

Alvin Hall,
Director, Management Analysis and Services Office, Centers for Disease Control and Prevention.

[FR Doc. 04–25536 Filed 11–17–04; 8:45 am]
BILLING CODE 4163–18–P

DEPARTMENT OF HEALTH AND HUMAN SERVICES

Centers for Disease Control and Prevention

Procedures and Costs for Use of the Research Data Center

AGENCY: National Center for Health Statistics, Centers for Disease Control and Prevention (CDC), Department of Health and Human Services (HHS).
ACTION: Notice and request for comments.

SUMMARY: This notice provides information about the Research Data Center (RDC) operated by the National Center for Health Statistics (NCHS) within the Centers for Disease Control and Prevention (CDC). The Research Data Center was established in 1998 to provide a mechanism whereby researchers can access detailed data files in a secure environment, without jeopardizing the confidentiality of respondents. Historically, the data files accessed in the RDC have consisted of NCHS survey data. RDC has recently begun accepting data files that were not produced from NCHS survey data. In order to assure that all data files are processed in a consistent manner, the original guidelines for accessing files in the RDC are being reviewed and revised as necessary. As part of the revision process, potential users are being given the opportunity to provide input on how the procedures of the RDC can best serve their research needs. This notice describes how to submit proposals requesting use of the data, mechanisms to access the RDC, requirements, use of outside data sets, costs for using the RDC, and other pertinent topics. We are seeking comments on these procedures and will post the final procedures on the NCHS Web site.

DATES: Submit comments on or before December 9, 2004.

ADDRESSES: Send comments concerning this notice to Ken Harris, National Center for Health Statistics, 3311 Toledo Road, Room 3210, Hyattsville, MD 20782, or e-mail to *kwharris@cdc.gov.*

FOR FURTHER INFORMATION CONTACT: Ken Harris at (301) 458–4262.

SUPPLEMENTARY INFORMATION:

Operational Procedures for Use of the Research Data Center; National Center for Health Statistics; Centers for Disease Control and Prevention

Table of Contents
Purpose
Background
Research Data Center—Operations
Submission of Research Proposals Using NCHS Data
Researcher—Supplied Data
General Requirements for Guest Researchers
General Requirements for Remote Access
Use of RDC/NCHS
Costs for Using the RDC
Disclosure Review Process
Appendix I—Examples of Data Available through the NCHS RDC
Appendix II—Requirements for the Release of NCHS Micro Data
Appendix III—Disallowed SAS Functions, Statements, and Procedures
Appendix IV—Project-Specific Requirements Vaccine Safety Datalink Files
Appendix V—Agreement Regarding Conditions of Access to Confidential Data in the Research Data Center of the National Center for Health Statistics
Appendix VI—Researcher Affidavit of Confidentiality

Operational Procedures for the Use of the Research Data Center, National Center for Health Statistics (NCHS); Centers for Disease Control and Prevention (CDC)

Purpose

This document provides information about the National Center for Health Statistics' (NCHS) Research Data Center (RDC), including how to submit proposals requesting use of data, mechanisms to access the RDC, requirements, use of outside data sets, costs for using the RDC, and other pertinent topics. The Guidelines pertain to use of data produced by NCHS and non-NCHS entities. If, after reading these guidelines, you have further questions, you may seek clarification through e-mail *(RDCA@cdc.gov)* or by contacting Ken Harris at (301) 458–4262 or by e-mail at *kwharris@cdc.gov.* The procedures described for use of the RDC are under constant review to improve RDC operations and to be responsive to changes in the environment that affect confidentiality protections. Please check the NCHS Web site or contact the RDC to determine if modifications have been made.

Background

In order to advance knowledge on the health and well-being of the nation and its health care system, NCHS and other organizational entities in the Department of Health and Human Services release statistical micro data containing health and related variables. These files allow outside researchers and analysts to develop statistics and conduct independent research. However, any release of data, whether micro data files or the results of statistical analyses, must be consistent with the confidentiality provisions under which the data were collected. For the case of data collected or obtained by NCHS, Section 308(d) of the Public Health Service Act (42 U.S.C. 242m(d)) and the NCHS Staff Manual on Confidentiality do not permit the release of data that are either identified or identifiable to persons outside of NCHS. In order to preserve privacy and confidentiality, details that might identify or facilitate the identification of persons and organizations participating in surveys and data systems are suppressed in published data products. Examples of data elements that might be abridged are geographic identifiers, details of sample design, and variables such as age or income that might exist in other databases.

Despite the wide dissemination of data through publications, CD–ROMs, etc., the inability to release files with, for instance, lower levels of geography, severely limits the utility of some data for research, policy, and programmatic purposes and sets a boundary on one of the goals of the U.S. Department of Health and Human Services, *i.e.*, to increase our capacity to provide state and local area estimates. In pursuit of this goal and in response to the research community's interest in restricted data, NCHS established the Research Data Center (RDC), a mechanism whereby researchers can access detailed data files in a secure environment, without jeopardizing the confidentiality of respondents. The RDC provides restricted access to NCHS data. The RDC also accepts outside data sets. Appendix I contains information about some of the data sets currently available in the RDC.

Special requirements for use of non-NCHS data can be found in Appendix IV, Project-Specific Requirements.

Authority: Sections 306 and 308 of the Public Health Service Act (42 U.S.C. 242k and 242m).

Research Data Center (RDC)—Operations

The NCHS RDC is a research facility located at the NCHS headquarters in Hyattsville, MD, where researchers meeting certain qualifications are allowed access, under strict supervision, to restricted statistical micro data files. To gain access to the RDC researchers must submit a proposal for review and approval. Researchers can use one of three access methods (see below): (1) Direct access through local computing resources in the RDC that accommodate visiting researchers; (2) a remote program submission system through which researchers can submit work to be done in the RDC with the output returned to them by e-mail, or (3) programming services for outside researchers provided by RDC staff (see below). In all three methods, confidential data files remain in the RDC where access to unit records is restricted, and output is inspected before it leaves the RDC.

As currently designed, the NCHS RDC facility in Hyattsville has four user workstations and a secure room for the RDC printer. In addition, there is office space for the RDC staff and long-term outside researchers.

The RDC computers have no electronic link either to the NCHS network, the CDC–NCHS mainframe, or the Internet. The RDC workstations consist of Pentium III 933 MHz computers running Windows 2000. There is sufficient storage on the workstations and the server for any confidential data. PC–SAS®, SUDAAN®, Watcom Fortran 77®, and Stata® are installed on the workstations, and additional programming/analytic languages can be added as needed.

The computers have been configured so that removable media such as floppy disks are inaccessible to users. All print output is routed to a central printer which is monitored by RDC staff while the RDC is open to external researchers. Further, the system's workstations are configured such that researchers are given read-only access to requested data files and can write only onto the local workstation's hard disk. These restrictions ensure that users cannot remove information that has not been subjected to a review for confidentiality.

The three methods of access to restricted data through the Data Center include:

(1) *Guest Researcher (on site)*—The researcher submits a research proposal to the RDC and, upon approval, conducts his/her research on site at NCHS in the RDC. RDC staff constructs the necessary data files before the guest researcher arrives and ensure that no restricted data leave the facility. Data from virtually all of the NCHS data collection systems may be made available through the RDC. Also available are data from other data collection systems.

PC–SAS®, SUDAAN®, Watcom Fortran 77®, and Stata® are installed on the RDC workstations. Other programming languages or data analysis packages can be made available with sufficient lead time.

Researchers may take the results of their analyses off-site only after disclosure review by NCHS RDC staff. Disclosure review consists of looking for tabular cells less than 5, tables with geographic variables in any dimension, models with geographic variables (or variables tantamount to geographic variables) as outcome variables, or case listings. In general, disclosure review is consistent with the guidelines published in the NCHS Staff Manual on Confidentiality (see Appendix II, Requirements for the Release of NCHS Micro Data Files).

(2) *Remote Access*—Users are able to electronically submit analytical computer programs using SAS as the programming language. After their proposals are approved, researchers are registered with the RDC remote access system and introduced to the procedures and programming limitations to be followed in accessing data. Researchers send programs to the RDC and receive output by e-mail. RDC staff prepares the requested data files which may consist of confidential data merged with user data. Both submitted programs and output undergo a programmed disclosure limitation review and are also subject to a manual review. Certain procedures and SAS® functions are not allowed (see Appendix II, Disallowed SAS® Functions, Statements, and Procedures for a complete list). For example, users cannot use PROC TABULATE or PROC IML, nor are functions allowed that are capable of producing listings of individual cases such as LIST and PRINT. Additionally, functions that may select individual cases are not allowed (R_, FIRST., LAST., and others). The output is scanned for cells containing less than five observations. If any are found, not only is that cell suppressed, but several additional cells will also be suppressed (complementary suppression). Alternatively, the researcher may be asked to revise and resubmit his/her analyses. The job log is also scanned with particular attention to certain types of error conditions that may spawn case listings. Some projects are not suitable for the remote access method. Stewards of the file/s in consultation with RDC staff make this determination.

(3) *RDC Staff-Assisted Research:* This is mainly useful for those planning to use statistical software programming languages other than SAS® or who are not able to travel to the RDC facility. Under this method, an approved researcher e-mails a statistical software program to the assigned RDC staff person who runs the program and, after disclosure review, provides the output to the researcher by e-mail. More extensive programming services are also available.

Each of the access methods outlined above has an associated cost which includes equipment and space rental, staff overhead, and setup. The staff overhead and setup include the time and resources necessary for monitoring progress, setting up equipment and data

APPENDIX G

files, disclosure limitation review, and file management. Since these reflect varying demands on resources, accurate cost estimates cannot be given without complete knowledge of the proposed research. In general, though, the setup fee is $500 per day of effort (see Costs of Using the RDC, below).

Submission of Research Proposals Using NCHS Data

Researchers must submit proposals that are detailed enough in their data specifications to permit RDC staff to easily determine what data elements are required. Prospective researchers are encouraged to check with RDC staff prior to writing their proposals to ensure that the data of interest can be made available to them. Researchers should develop their proposals in a way that facilitates the ability of the RDC staff to create the analytic files required by the project. Proposals should be explicit regarding the variables needed as well as any case selection required. Only those data items required to conduct the proposed analyses will be included in the analytic data file and the proposals should address why the requested data are needed for the proposed study. Overly large and complex projects or poorly defined projects will require extensive communication between RDC staff and the researchers proposing the project, and this can cause the process to move slowly. Work to prepare data files can be accomplished most expeditiously if large, complex projects are subdivided into manageable parts and requested data are clearly defined.

Researchers wishing to link data in the RDC with external data should provide the external data to RDC staff in advance of their entry to and use of the RDC (a minimum of 7 days prior to the approved date for access to the RDC).

The RDC expects that all researchers will adhere to established standards and principles for carrying out statistical research and analyses. Researchers must conduct only those analyses which received approval. Failure to comply will result in cancellation of the research activity and potential disbarment from future research activities in the RDC. In the case where Institutional Review Board (IRB) approval is required to conduct research, RDC staff will notify relevant IRBs of infringements of protocol approvals.

Appendix IV (Project-Specific Requirements) contains information on submitting a research proposal requesting use of data other than those produced by NCHS. The format detailed below pertains specifically to use of NCHS data. If no project specific requirements are provided for non-NCHS data, the format below is to be used.

(1) The research proposal must contain the following information:
  A. Cover letter.
  B. Project Title.
  C. Abstract: approximately 100–300 words summarizing the project.
  D. Full personal identification, institutional affiliation, mailing addresses (including overnight express mail address), phone, and e-mail address. Applicants who are students must append a letter from the department chair or advisor stating that the applicant is a student working under the direction of the department.
  E. Dates of proposed tenure at the RDC (or use of the remote access system). Proposals requesting remote access should include an appendix describing the computer and e-mail account that will receive output as well as the security provisions established for them.
  F. Source of funding for the proposed project.
  G. Background of study:
    1. Key study questions or hypotheses.
    2. Public health benefits.
  H. A summary of the data requirements for the proposed research along with an explanation of why the data are needed for the proposed study.
    1. Identification of cases to be included in the analytic file.
    2. Identification of variables to be included in the analytic file.
    3. Data to be supplied by the researcher and merged with NCHS or other data.
    4. A description of why publicly available data are insufficient.
  I. Methods for the study:
    1. Analytic strategy and statistical methods to be used.
    2. Software requirements (currently, PC–SAS® for Windows®, Stata®, SUDAAN®, LIMDEP®, HLM®, SPSS®, and Watcom Fortran 77® are available in the RDC; other languages can be made available with sufficient lead time).
  J. A description of the output that the researcher intends to have reviewed for non-disclosure. This should include table shells, model equations, or test statistics of any output that the researcher plans to remove from the RDC. This will help the reviewers to determine the risk of disclosure.
  K. Appendices.
    1. A current resume or Curriculum Vitae for each person who will participate in the research activity. Resumes or CVs must specify nationality.
    2. A letter from student applicant's department chair or academic advisor stating that student is working under the direction of the department.
    3. A data dictionary: a complete listing of the specific data requested—data system, files, years, cases, variables, matching or linking variables, etc.
    4. A data dictionary for researcher-supplied data, if any, to be merged with the confidential data. This includes identifying the source of the data, variable names, variable codes or ranges, file layout, number of records, and restrictions on NCHS use of the data (currently the RDC policy prohibits release of merged data to anyone other than the prospective researcher).
    5. A description of the computer and e-mail system to be used to receive output from the remote access system as well as the security provisions established for them.

Portions of doctoral proposals or grant applications with appropriate modifications may suffice for the research proposal.

Proposals to use the Research Data Center should be sent to:
Research Data Center, National Center for Health Statistics, 3311 Toledo Road, Suite 4113, Hyattsville, MD 20782, *RDCA@cdc.gov*.

Upon receipt, the Research Proposal will be evaluated by a review committee convened for that purpose. The Proposal Review Committee consists of (at minimum) the director of the NCHS RDC, the RDC staff liaison, the NCHS Confidentiality Officer, and the director (or designee) of the NCHS data division whose data are requested in the proposal. Proposals for use of non-NCHS data undergo review as determined by the steward/s of those data.

(2) The following criteria apply to proposal review for projects requesting use of NCHS data:
  A. Scientific and technical feasibility of the project;
  B. Availability of resources at the RDC;
  C. Risk of disclosure of restricted information; and
  D. For projects using NCHS data, whether the proposed project is in accordance with the mission of the NCHS to provide statistical information that will guide actions and policies to improve the health of the American people.

Researchers should note that approval of their application does not constitute endorsement by NCHS of the substantive, methodological, theoretical, or policy relevance or merit of the proposed research. NCHS approval only

VACCINE SAFETY RESEARCH

constitutes a judgment that this research, as described in the application, is not an illegal use of the requested data file and that there is high probability that the project can be successfully done in the RDC.

Researcher-Supplied Data

The RDC allows researchers to supply their own data to be linked with RDC data sets to create merged data sets that will be stored in the RDC. The researcher-supplied data may consist of proprietary data collected and "owned" by the researcher or other publicly available data obtained by the researcher such as census data. Researchers MUST provide RDC staff with complete documentation of any data proposed to be merged with RDC data. Researchers expecting to use merged files are responsible for interacting with RDC staff to ensure that their data can be merged with the data resident at the RDC and the format of the data is consistent with the RDC data. The RDC will accept user data files in SAS®, Stata®, or ASCII® format (flat files) with variables either column-delimited or column-specific. Other formats may also be proposed. RDC staff prior to the arrival of the researcher will do the merging of researcher-supplied data with RDC data sets. Identifying information in linking fields will be removed after the merge and will not be made available to the researchers.

Owners or stewards of RDC data sets make the determination of whether and how the resultant merged files would be made available to other researchers. For RDC files that are owned by NCHS, this determination is made by the owners of the researcher-supplied data that will be merged with the NCHS owned RDC files. For files that are NOT owned by NCHS, the determination is made by the stewards or owners of the RDC files. The owners of these files can require that any merged files be made available to all interested researchers or allow this determination to be made by the owners of the researcher supplied data.

The RDC periodically creates and maintains backup copies of all computer files. Backup files are stored in a secure storage area accessible by RDC staff only, although they may be made available to researchers who need to return for additional analyses. These backup files will contain user-supplied data as well as the merged files. These backup files will be destroyed only upon the written request of the user.

General Requirements for Guest Researchers

1. Researchers must work under the supervision of RDC staff and only during normal working hours (Monday–Friday, 8:30 a.m.–5 p.m.). Admittance to the RDC will be limited to the researchers whose names are included in the Research Proposal (Section D). Researchers will be required to show photo identification before admittance. A maximum of 3 collaborating researchers can sit at a computer station in the RDC.

2. Computers will be pre-loaded with the approved datasets by NCHS staff approximately one day prior to the external researcher's use of the RDC. Once the analysis is completed, NCHS staff will remove the datasets from the RDC computer.

3. Guest researchers must be able to conduct their analyses with the software specified in their research proposal.

4. External researchers are not allowed to bring documents, manuals, books, etc., that may enable them to identify and disclose confidential information they access in the RDC. Neither are they allowed to bring into the RDC cell phones, pagers, or other devices which would enable them to communicate with persons outside of the RDC.

5. All logs will be printed or electronically archived and will be kept by NCHS. NCHS will retain only the programs and procedures run by external researchers. The logs will not include results from their research.

6. All computer output generated by statistical programs and all hand-written notes based on such computer output are subject to disclosure review by NCHS staff before removal from the RDC. Output is restricted to summary tables of geographic or patient-level data (e.g., line listings of diagnoses by study identifier will be prohibited).

7. Guest researchers may not save output, files, or programs to transportable electronic media. RDC staff can copy output or programs to transportable media, if requested.

8. Researchers proposing multiple analyses that employ multiple data sets will have access to only one dataset at a time. Under no circumstances will researchers be permitted any opportunity to merge datasets on their own.

General Requirements for Remote Access

1. Researchers must register an e-mail address that is credibly secure. Although programs can be sent to the RDC from any address, results will always be returned to the registered e-mail address.

2. Data requests must be in the form of SAS® programs (Version 8.2). However, certain SAS® commands/statements are not allowed through remote access. A list of such commands/statements is included in Appendix III. This list is periodically reviewed and may be modified as necessary. The SAS® program must be in plain ASCII® format.

3. During the first week of registration, researchers' data requests are executed in a manual mode, requiring RDC staff to review the program and resulting output before its release. During this period, remote access is available only during normal working hours. After the first week, researchers may submit data requests any time (day or night) and receive prompt response, except when the CDC e-mail system is down or when the remote access system is taken off-line for maintenance.

4. The remote access system does not allow users to write permanent datasets in its disk space. Jobs that attempt to create permanent datasets or files are flagged, terminated, and an error message is sent to the researcher.

5. The remote access system limits researchers' time and storage. No single program is allowed more than one hour to complete execution or to generate output in access of 1.5 MB.

6. With one exception, macros are not allowed through the remote access system. The exception, GLIMIX®, requires special permission.

Use of the RDC

In order to get access to restricted data files in the RDC, researchers must include in their proposals a signed "Agreement Regarding Conditions of Access to Confidential Data in the Research Data Center for the National Center for Health Statistics." (Appendix V) All researchers participating on an approved project must sign the agreement—which clearly states the penalties for violating the conditions of agreement. In addition, each researcher must sign an "Affidavit of Confidentiality." (Appendix VI) The RDC reserves the right to terminate any project at any time that it deems that an investigator's actions will compromise confidentiality or ethical standards of behavior in a research environment.

Statistical micro data files are collections of data from individual units such as persons or providers. Statistical agencies world wide are bound by ethical and legal requirements to preserve the privacy of individual respondents and the confidentiality of data provided to the agency by them or otherwise pertaining to them. As mentioned earlier, confidentiality protection at NCHS is governed by Section 308(d) of the Public Health

APPENDIX G   137

Service Act (42 U.S.C. 242m). This section states that:

No information, if an establishment or person supplying the information or described in it is identifiable, obtained in the course of activities undertaken or supported under section 304, 306, or 307 may be used for any purpose other than the purpose for which it was supplied unless such establishment or person has consented (as determined under regulations of the Secretary) to its use for such other purpose and in the case of information obtained in the course of health statistical or epidemiological activities under section 304 or 306, such information may not be published or released in other form if the particular establishment or person supplying the information or described in it is identifiable unless such establishment or person has consented (as determined under regulations of the Secretary) to its publication or release in other form.

Having read and familiarized themselves with the Researcher Affidavit of Confidentiality, including Section 308(d) of the Public Health Service Act (42 U.S.C. 242m) (see below), researchers agree:

1. To make no copies of any files or portions of files to which they are granted access except those authorized by NCHS Research Data Center staff.

2. To return to RDC staff all NCHS restricted materials with which they may be provided during the conduct of their research at NCHS and other materials as requested.

3. Not to use ANY technique in an attempt to learn the identity of any person, establishment, or sampling unit not identified on public use data files.

4. To hold in strictest confidence the identification of any establishment or individual that may be inadvertently revealed in any documents or discussion, or analysis. Such inadvertent identification revealed in their analyses will be immediately brought to the attention of RDC staff.

5. Not to remove any printouts, electronic files, documents, or media until they have been scanned for disclosure risk by RDC staff.

6. Not to remove from NCHS any written notes pertaining to the identification of any establishment, individual, or geographic area that may be revealed in the conduct of their research at NCHS.

7. To the inspection of any material they may bring to or remove from the NCHS Research Data Center.

8. To comport themselves in a manner consistent with principles and standards appropriate to a scientific research establishment.

Appendix V Agreement Regarding Conditions of Access to Confidential Data in the Research Data Center of the National Center for Health Statistics, signed by all investigators on the project, must be submitted with the initial proposal.

Deliberate violation of any of these conditions may result in cancellation of the data access, and the researcher may be escorted from the premises by the duly authorized Federal protection service on duty at NCHS. The researcher may also be barred from any future use of the RDC upon review and determination by the Director of NCHS that this is necessary to protect the integrity and confidentiality of the RDC.

The RDC technical monitor will perform a disclosure review and must provide approval to the researcher before removal of any data from the RDC, whether it is in electronic or paper form. Any violation by the researcher may be punishable by fine or imprisonment for up to 5 years or both under Title 18 U.S.C. 1001.

As noted above, the RDC contains work stations with computers pre-loaded by NCHS staff with the requested dataset(s) to be analyzed with statistical software. External researchers must schedule time for use of the RDC, pay the appropriate user fees, and abide by the standard practices of the RDC. Among the requirements is a restriction on equipment that can be brought into the RDC, signing agreements to maintain confidentiality, and submitting to review of all results for any potential breaches in confidentiality.

Costs for Using the RDC

Time in the RDC can be scheduled in increments ranging from a consecutive 2-day minimum to a consecutive 10-day maximum. Extensions can be negotiated with RDC staff subject to scheduling requirements. Scheduling time at the RDC is on a first-come, first-served basis.

Researchers using the NCHS RDC will be charged for space and equipment rental and staff time necessary for supervision, disclosure limitation review, maintenance of computer facilities (including both hardware and software), and the creation and maintenance of data files required by the researcher. The cost per project (or creation of an analytic file) is given in the table below:

Guest Researcher (on site)	$200 per day (2-day minimum).
Remote Access	$500 per month for files with less than 130,000 records.
	$1,000 per month for files with 130,000 records or more.
	$500 per year for selected standard files.*

*There are selected files that have been developed for repeat and multiple users which require minimal set up procedures and involve minimal content changes to the file when preparing for different users. For that reason, charges for accessing these files are considerably less expensive than the regular fees. Two files fall under this category: the contextual data file for the National Survey of Family Growth (NSFG–CDF) and the Polio file for the National Health Interview Survey (NHIS–Polio). The cost of accessing standard files of this type will be published as the files are developed.

There is a minimum setup charge of $500 per day for new file creation. An additional $500 per day is charged as needed for file creations and for special handling, such as the merging of additional data or creating custom file formats.

More complex projects may require discussion between the researcher and RDC staff to determine the cost of file creation. Researchers are encouraged to develop their proposals in a way that facilitates the ability of the RDC staff to create the analytic files required by the project. Proposals should be explicit regarding the variables needed as well as any case selection required. Overly large and complex projects will require extensive communication between RDC staff and the researchers proposing the project, and this can cause the process to move slowly. Work to prepare data files can be accomplished most expeditiously if large, complex projects are subdivided into manageable parts.

Payment is expected in advance of the use of the RDC. A cashier's check or money order made payable to NCHS RDC must be received seven business days prior to the start date scheduled for use of the RDC. Payments should be mailed to: NCHS RDC, Attn: RDC Director, 3311 Toledo Road, Suite 4113, Hyattsville, MD 20782.

Disclosure Review Process

The disclosure review process in the RDC is centered on a rigorously conducted research base. Briefly, RDC staff, either independently or in collaboration with staff from other areas of the NCHS, other government agencies, and non-governmental researchers, conduct research into the use of technological and statistical advances to develop and refine additional methods to access restricted data such as the use of the internet or encrypted data, assessment of disclosure risk through statistical and automated procedures, and the use of disclosure limitation methodologies (*e.g.*, statistical noise) to enable the release of otherwise restricted data files. The results of these research activities are applied to disclosure review activities in the RDC.

Researchers may take the results of their analyses off-site after disclosure review by RDC staff. Disclosure review consists of looking for tabular cells less than 5, tables with geographic variables in any dimension, models with geographic variables (or variables tantamount to geographic variables) as outcome variables, or line listings. In general, disclosure review is consistent with the guidelines published in the NCHS Staff Manual on Confidentiality (see Appendix II, Requirements for the Release of Micro Data).

RDC staff review data summaries to assure maintenance of respondent confidentiality. In no case may any table contain cells with fewer than 5 observations. If found, these small cells are suppressed, generally by obliterating the cell. To assure that small cells cannot be calculated from the other cells in the same row or column, staff makes illegible best fits for the rows and columns corresponding to the small cell. Once disclosure review is completed, researchers receive a photocopy of the final tabulations.

RDC staff when reviewing cross-tabulations for small cell use the following procedures:

1. Shred all tables having fewer than five total observations (table total);
2. Shred all tables having fewer than five observations in each cell ;
3. If the table passes the first two criteria, RDC staff will review the table one row at a time;
4. Make illegible all counts and percents for cells with four or fewer observations;
5. If one row cell is <5, that cell and at least one other row cell will be suppressed; if two or more row cells are each <5, each will be suppressed, but the row total need not be suppressed because the suppressed row cells cannot be determined;
6. If one column cell is <5, that cell and at least one other column cell will be suppressed; if two or more column cells are each <5, each will be suppressed, but the column total need not be suppressed because the suppressed column cells cannot be determined;
7. Row (or column) total is suppressed ONLY if it (*i.e.*, total) is <5; since the cells that are <5 (row or column as appropriate) are suppressed, user cannot determine their values by knowing the row (or column) total.

RDC staff will use best practices in determining whether data are identifiable and will be conservative in their decisions. RDC decisions are final and not subject to negotiation by researchers.

Publication

For NCHS files, any published material derived from the data should acknowledge NCHS as the source and should include a disclaimer that credits any analyses, interpretations, or conclusions reached by the author (recipient of the file) to that author and not to NCHS, which is responsible only for the initial data. Researchers who want to publish a technical description of the data should make a reasonable effort to ensure that the description is consistent with that published by NCHS.

Appendix I—Examples of NCHS Data Available Through the NCHS RDC

National Health Interview Survey—Data from the core and supplements for survey years 1987–2002 are available for merging user-supplied data at the state and county levels (note that RDC users do not have access to county FIPS codes; these are replaced with randomly assigned dummy codes). Additionally, state data files may be made available for analysis and reporting.

National Survey of Family Growth— Contextual Data File—The 1995 NSFG has available sets of contextual variables at the state, county, census tract, and block-group levels for the residence of the respondents in 1990, 1993, and 1995.

Third National Health and Nutrition Examination Survey (1988–1994)—Data from NHANES III are available with state and county identifiers (there are restrictions on the use and reporting of geographic units).

NCHS survey data, including vital statistics, Longitudinal Study on Aging, and other data files with restricted information (sample design information, lower levels of geography, etc.) can be made available as requested and needed.

Appendix II—Requirements for the Release of NCHS Micro Data Files

The following rules apply to all files released by NCHS which contain any information about individual persons or establishments, except where the supplier of information was told, prior to his giving the information, that the information would be made public:

A. Before any new or revised micro data files are published, they, together with their full documentation, must be approved for publication by the Confidentiality Officer who will rely upon assistance from the NCHS Disclosure Review Board in reaching decisions.

B. The file must not contain any detailed information about the subject that could facilitate identification and that is not essential for research purposes (*e.g.*, exact date of the subject's birth, excessive detail for occupation, extreme values of income and age, detailed race or ethnicity for small and highly visible groups—and other characteristics that would make an individual or establishment easier to identify). It is recommended that the following be consulted concerning possible techniques that would permit the maximum amount of information to be released consistent with sound principles of statistical disclosure limitation: The Confidentiality and Data Access Committee's Checklist on Disclosure Potential of Data *(http:// www.fcsm.gov/committees/cdac/ checklist_799.doc)* and Statistical Policy Working Paper 22, Report on Statistical Disclosure Limitation Methodology. Office of Information and Regulatory Affairs, Office of Management and Budget *(http:// www.fcsm.gov/working-papers/wp22.html)*.

C. Geographic places that have fewer than 100,000 people are not to be identified on the file. Depending upon the statistical structure of a file and other circumstances, a higher figure may be employed. It is the responsibility of the program proposing the data release to determine the disclosure risk associated with the proposed minimum size of geographic areas to be identified.

D. Characteristics of an area are not to appear on the file if they would uniquely identify an area of fewer than 100,000 people (*e.g.*, a variable describing the size of a Metropolitan Area in which a respondent was interviewed providing for a category of fewer than 100,000 in a file where Region is also provided).

E. Information on the drawing of the sample which might assist in identifying a respondent must not be released outside the Center. Thus, the identities of primary sampling units are not to be made available outside the Research Data Center except in limited circumstances as approved by the Confidentiality Officer. When such circumstances require the disclosure of the identity of areas in which data collection activities take place, the survey manager must insure that all information for this survey proposed for release takes into account the greater risk of identification because of this exception. The decision as to whether PSU identities are to be made public should be made before data are collected and plans for data release finalized.

Appendix III—Disallowed SAS® Functions, Statements, and Procedures

The list below is used by the RDC remote access system to scan user-submitted programs for functions, statements, and procedures that may result in an unauthorized disclosure. Any user-submitted program that contains one or more of these

APPENDIX G

keywords is automatically rejected, and the user is asked to correct the problem and resubmit the program. Because the remote access system is an automated system, the RDC does not and cannot make any exceptions. This list may change pending development of additional methodologies.

r_word
add
print
obs
firstobs
first.
last.
&
%
nocol
report
pctn
pctsum
tabulate
iml
nofreq
nocum
browse
editor
summary
list
put
file
r_
plot
PROC DATASET:
-Copy
-Delete
-Rename
-Repair
-Append
-List
Compress
Pointobs
multi part data set names

In addition to the above disallowed statements and functions, users of the remote access system cannot use any statements or functions that write permanent data files to the hard disk.

Appendix IV—Project-Specific Requirements

Vaccine Safety Datalink (VSD) Project

The VSD was established to allow the Centers for Disease Control and Prevention (CDC) to carefully monitor vaccine safety in the United States. The VSD, a large-linked database, contains medical and immunization information on more than six million people annually. Information available in the database includes basic demographic information, managed care organization (MCO) enrollment, dates of vaccination, and medical visits. The VSD is a collaborative project involving CDC and several large MCOs. Information from the VSD is used by CDC to conduct vaccine safety studies.

Recognition of the need for improved monitoring of vaccine safety prompted the CDC to initiate the VSD project in 1990. This project currently involves partnerships with MCOs to continually monitor vaccine safety. All vaccines administered within a MCO are recorded and include vaccine type, date of vaccination, concurrent vaccinations (those given during the same visit), the manufacturer, lot number and injection site. Medical visits are also recorded which can be used to monitor for potential adverse events resulting from immunization. The VSD project allows for planned vaccine safety studies as well as timely investigations of emerging hypotheses. At present, the VSD project is examining potential associations between vaccines and a number of serious conditions. Data from the VSD also are used to test new vaccine safety hypotheses that result from the medical literature, signals from the Vaccine Adverse Events Reporting System (VAERS), changes in the immunization schedule, the introduction of new vaccines, or recommendations from the Institute of Medicine (IOM) and Advisory Committee on Immunization Practices (ACIP) recommendations. This project is a powerful and cost-effective tool for the on-going evaluation of vaccine safety. It should be noted that the MCOs, as owners of the data, have broad decision-making authority over data release, as specified in CDC's contract with America's Health Insurance Plans (AHIP). In addition, MCOs have a recognized need and right to protect proprietary data.

In August 2002, CDC's National Immunization Program (NIP) and its managed care partners created a data sharing program to allow limited access to VSD data through the NCHS RDC with confidentiality protection under Sec. 308(d) of the Public Health Service Act (42 U.S.C. 242m). Proposals requesting use of VSD data undergo a review by the MCOs' Institutional Review Board(s) (MCO IRB) in addition to a review by RDC staff. After approval of their research proposal and payment of fees for the associated costs, researchers are able to independently analyze data from the VSD.

Two types of VSD data may be accessed at the RDC by an external researcher:

1. Analytic datasets created from the VSD data files that reside at CDC to conduct new vaccine safety studies:

The VSD data files are comprised of several separate data sets derived from computerized data sources from seven participating VSD MCOs. The VSD data files contain data through December 31, 2000 and include information such as vaccinations, hospital discharge and other diagnoses, and demographic characteristics. With these data, an external researcher may conduct a new vaccine safety study in order to test his/her vaccine safety hypothesis. The external researcher may request only the variables that are found in the VSD data Files (as listed in the data dictionary).

To assist researchers, CDC makes available at its Web site: (1) A list of recommended scientific references relevant to conducting research using large linked databases such as the VSD data files and (2) a data dictionary that lists all the variables contained in the VSD data files available for new vaccine safety research (http://www.cdc.gov/nip/vacsafe/vsd/default.htm#data).

Proposals for analyses of new vaccine safety studies using data from the VSD data files should include only those specific variables that are needed to conduct the proposed analyses, including a brief explanation with justification for use of these variables.

Data contained in the VSD data files have been created from MCO administrative data which are not solely collected for the purpose of scientific research. It should be noted then that potential data discrepancies and varying degrees of data quality that are specific to such types of data do exist and typically are not resolvable with data that are available in the RDC.

2. Final datasets from published VSD studies:

External researchers who would like to perform a reanalysis of a published VSD study performed by VSD investigators may request the final dataset for the specific study they wish to re-analyze. Data collected for the final datasets of the published studies may include additional variables not listed in the data dictionary that is referenced above; therefore, the RDC will provide the external researcher with the necessary data dictionary for the requested dataset(s). No additional source or "raw" data are available for reanalysis of published VSD studies.

In general, VSD studies published after August 2002 are available for reanalysis. However, since many studies were published prior to the establishment of the CDC data sharing policy, some of the earlier published VSD study datasets may not be available for re-analysis for the following reasons:

• Some IRBs mandate that datasets be destroyed after research is completed.
• Principal investigator may no longer be affiliated with VSD or the collaborating MCOs; therefore, the location of the dataset is unknown.
• Rapidly changing technology can mean that data are on obsolete media.

Following receipt of a proposal for a reanalysis, the RDC will verify that the data variables requested from the published study are available. If these data are not available (for one or more of the reasons stated above), the RDC will notify the external researcher. Documentation for variables and datasets used in VSD studies completed after August 2002 are maintained according to the CDC data sharing policy regarding archival of data that are available on the Web at http://www.cdc.gov/od/ads/pol-385.htm.

All proposals requesting use of VSD data should contain the following information:

A. Project Title.
B. Name of proposed investigator and collaborators (RDC rules limit number of persons at a work station to 3 at a time).
C. Name of point of contact, address, telephone number, and e-mail address.
D. Summary of proposed study (*i.e.*, background, reasons for conducting the study, public health benefits).
E. Specific hypothesis for new vaccine safety studies to be investigated or title of published VSD study to be reanalyzed.
F. Proposed methodology for new vaccine safety studies or the specification of the methods used in published VSD studies:
 1. Definition of the study population of interest and type of study to be conducted:
  a. Descriptive studies: specify the variables and values for those variables to be used to select the study population.
  b. Case-control studies: specify criteria for cases and controls.
  c. Cohort studies: specify criteria for the exposed and unexposed population.
  d. For all new vaccine safety studies, please include the following information as

part of the definition of the study population of interest:
  i. Adult or Pediatric data (0–17 or 18+).
  ii. Study years of interest (i.e. 199X–2000). Please note the study years available vary by HMO site.
  iii. How the study population will be selected from the VSD data files based on available fields in the VSD data dictionary.
  2. Specification of the variables that will be required including:
    a. Exposures: Specific criteria defining exposures based on the VSD data dictionary should be included. For instance, specific vaccines given within 14 days of the outcome of interest.
    b. Outcomes: Specific criteria defining those outcomes based on the VSD data dictionary should be included. For instance, specific ICD–9 codes for outcomes of interest and type of health care encounter (hospitalization, outpatient encounter, emergency room visit).
    c. Person Time or Enrollment: Specify criteria to determine calculation of person time, follow-up time, or MCO enrollment restrictions.
    d. Confounding or control variables, including:
      1. Demographic information.
      2. Pre-existing or co-morbid conditions.
      3. Concurrent vaccinations.
      4. MCO Site.
    e. Other required variables to perform the proposed analysis.
  G. Proposed analytic strategies.

The RDC staff will notify the external researcher whether his/her proposal is complete and whether the requested variables are available. If all the requested data variables can be located for the proposed new vaccine safety studies or proposed reanalysis, review of the proposal by the appropriate MCO IRBs takes place. In compliance with federal law and regulations, access by external researchers to a portion of the VSD data files or to datasets from VSD published studies requires review and approval by the appropriate IRBs of the relevant MCOs. The MCO IRBs have the responsibility to protect the confidentiality and privacy of their members' medical records and to adhere to the rules and regulations applicable to their respective institution(s). Consequently, each of the MCO IRBs must review any request for access to the VSD data files that contain information on its MCO members. Any appeal by the requestor of an IRB decision must follow the national, federal procedures for IRBs. CDC is not involved in the MCO IRB process at any time. General information pertaining to the rules and regulations of IRB submission can be found at http://www.cdc.gov/od/ads/hsr2.html/.

Submission of Proposals to MCO IRBs

Review of a proposal submitted by an external researcher by a MCO IRB does not imply that CDC approves or endorses the external researcher's proposed research. IRB applications may require a more detailed description of the proposed vaccine safety study and may vary according to individual IRB requirements. Furthermore, various IRBs may have different time lines for submission of proposals for review. Each IRB may have specific policies or requirements for data sharing that have not been adopted by the other MCO IRBs. These policies may include required collaboration with an MCO investigator, fees associated with the IRB review process, or differing criteria for the IRB review process.

MCO IRBs will use their established procedures and time lines to review the proposed research and to consider any appeals. As a rule, IRBs attempt to inform researchers as to the status of their proposals. Approval for access to MCO data contained within the VSD data files does not indicate approval for obtaining additional data contained within the MCO's member medical records or elsewhere, if such data are not contained within the VSD data files that reside in the RDC.

For new vaccine safety studies, it is possible that an external researcher will receive approval for access to VSD data from some, but not all, relevant IRBs. If this occurs, then the dataset(s) needed to conduct the new vaccine safety study will still be created, but only with data from the MCOs whose IRBs approved access. VSD data sets for new vaccine safety studies must contain data from two or more MCOs' data. Access will not be provided to data from only one MCO. For reanalysis of a published VSD study, all relevant IRBs from the MCOs that participated in the published study must approve the proposal for reanalysis; therefore if one or more IRBs do not approve access to VSD data used in the published study, the final dataset cannot be provided.

Once the external researcher has received a response from all of the appropriate IRBs, the RDC will begin the process of creating or formatting the approved dataset(s). The RDC will not create or prepare the dataset(s) until it receives copies of all final IRB dispositions.

Publication of Research Using VSD Data

When an external researcher has completed his/her work at the RDC and wishes to publish research results and findings using VSD data, there are specific requirements that must be followed:
• External researchers are required to submit a copy of these data sharing guidelines with any manuscript submitted to a journal.
• External researchers are required to submit (to the journal) a copy of the Confidentiality Agreement he/she signed prior to conducting research at the RDC.
• Disclaimers must be included in the manuscript which state:
  The research was conducted using data from the Vaccine Safety Datalink Project, through the data sharing program at the Centers for Disease Control and Prevention.
• Any published material using VSD data must acknowledge CDC as the original data source.
• Additionally, disclaimers must be included that state:
  The analysis, interpretations, and conclusions are the responsibility of the authors and do not represent the views and opinions of the CDC, the Federal Government, or the managed care organization providing the data.

Appendix V—Agreement Regarding Conditions of Access to Confidential Data in the Research Data Center of the National Center for Health Statistics

I _____ (please print name) am aware that the information contained in the (name of data file) has been provided to NCHS in accordance with the provisions of Section 308(d) of the Public Health Service Act (42 U.S.C. 242m), with the assurance that it will be used only for health statistical reporting and analysis and will not be published or released in identifiable form. I am also aware that I can be held legally liable for any harm incurred by individuals or establishments who have provided or are described in the information contained in the above work files to which I will have access.

Having read and familiarized myself with the Researcher Affidavit of Confidentiality, including Section 308(d) of the Public Health Service Act (42 U.S.C. 242m) (attached), I agree:

1. To make no copies of any files or portions of files to which I am granted access except those authorized by NCHS Research Data Center staff.
2. To return to RDC staff all NCHS restricted materials with which I may be provided during the conduct of my research at NCHS and other materials as requested.
3. Not to use ANY technique in an attempt to learn the identity of any person, establishment, or sampling unit not identified on public use data files.
4. To hold in strictest confidence the identification of any establishment or individual that may be inadvertently revealed in any documents or discussion, or analysis. Such inadvertent identification revealed in my analysis will be immediately brought to the attention of RDC staff.
5. Not to remove any printouts, electronic files, documents, or media until they have been scanned for disclosure risk by RDC staff.
6. Not to remove from NCHS any written notes pertaining to the identification of any establishment, individual, or geographic area that may be revealed in the conduct of my research at NCHS.
7. To the inspection of any material I may bring to or remove from the NCHS Research Data Center.
8. To comport myself in a manner consistent with the principles and standards appropriate to a scientific research establishment.

Deliberate violation of any of these conditions may result in cancellation of the data access agreement, and the researcher may be escorted from the premises by the duly authorized Federal protection service on duty at NCHS. The researcher may also be barred from any future use of the RDC upon review and determination by the Director of NCHS that this is necessary to protect the integrity and confidentiality of the RDC.

Researcher's Signature _____

Date _____

NCHS Witness _____

Date _____

APPENDIX G

141

67592   **Federal Register** / Vol. 69, No. 222 / Thursday, November 18, 2004 / Notices

Appendix VI—Researcher Affidavit of Confidentiality

I certify that no confidential data or information viewed or otherwise obtained while I am a researcher in the National Center for Health Statistics (NCHS) Research Data Center (RDC) will be removed from NCHS. Further, I understand that NCHS will perform a disclosure review and must provide approval to me before I remove any data from the RDC, whether they are in electronic or paper form. I acknowledge NCHS Confidentiality Statute, Sec. 308(d) of the Public Health Service Act (42 U.S.C. 242m) stated below and fully understand my legal obligations to NCHS to protect all confidential data. Further, I understand that any violation may be punishable by fine or imprisonment for up to 5 years or both under Title 18 U.S.C. 1001.

NCHS Confidentiality Statute—No information, if an establishment or person supplying the information or described in it is identifiable, obtained in the course of activities undertaken or supported under section 304, 306, or 307 may be used for any purpose other than the purpose for which it was supplied unless such establishment or person has consented (as determined under regulations of the Secretary) to its use for such other purpose and in the case of information obtained in the course of health statistical or epidemiological activities under section 304 or 306, such information may not be published or released in other form if the particular establishment or person supplying the information or described in it is identifiable unless such establishment or person has consented (as determined under regulations of the Secretary) to its publication or release in other form.

Title 18 U.S.C. 1001—Deliberately making a false statement in any matter within the jurisdiction of any Department or Agency of the Federal Government violates Title 18 U.S.C. 1001 and is punishable by a fine or up to 5 years in prison or both.

Researcher's Signature

Date

NCHS Witness

Date

Dated: November 9, 2004.

James D. Seligman,
Associate Director for Program Services, Centers for Disease Control and Prevention.

[FR Doc. 04–25537 Filed 11–17–04; 8:45 am]

BILLING CODE 4163–18–P

DEPARTMENT OF HEALTH AND HUMAN SERVICES

Food and Drug Administration

Oncologic Drugs Advisory Committee; Notice of Meeting

AGENCY: Food and Drug Administration, HHS.

ACTION: Notice.

This notice announces a forthcoming meeting of a public advisory committee of the Food and Drug Administration (FDA). The meeting will be open to the public.

Name of Committee: Oncologic Drugs Advisory Committee.

General Function of the Committee: To provide advice and recommendations to the agency on FDA's regulatory issues.

Date and Time: The meeting will be held on December 1, 2004, from 8 a.m. to 5 p.m.

Location: Holiday Inn, Kennedy/Adams Ballroom, 8777 Georgia Ave., Silver Spring, MD.

Contact Person: Johanna M. Clifford, Center for Drug Evaluation and Research (HFD–21), Food and Drug Administration, 5600 Fishers Lane, (for express delivery, 5630 Fishers Lane, rm. 1093) Rockville, MD 20857, 301–827–7001, Fax: 301–827–6776, e-mail: *cliffordj@cder.fda.gov*, or FDA Advisory Committee Information Line, 1–800–741–8138 (301–443–0572 in the Washington, DC area), code 3014512542. Please call the Information Line for up-to-date information on this meeting.

Agenda: The committee will discuss these items: (1) New drug application (NDA) 21–673, proposed trade name CLOLAR (clofarabine) Ilex Products, Inc., proposed indication for the treatment of pediatric patients 1 to 21 years old with refractory or relapsed acute leukemias, and (2) NDA 21–600, proposed trade name MARQIBO (vincristine sulfate liposome injection) Inex Pharmaceuticals Corp., proposed indication for the treatment of patients with aggressive non-Hodgkin's lymphoma previously treated with at least two combination chemotherapy regimens.

Procedure: Interested persons may present data, information, or views, orally or in writing, on issues pending before the committee. Written submissions may be made to the contact person by November 23, 2004. Oral presentations from the public will be scheduled between approximately 10:30 a.m. and 11 a.m., and between approximately 2:30 p.m. and 3 p.m. Time allotted for each presentation may be limited. Those desiring to make formal oral presentations should notify the contact person before November 23, 2004, and submit a brief statement of the general nature of the evidence or arguments they wish to present, the names and addresses of proposed participants, and an indication of the approximate time requested to make their presentation.

Persons attending FDA's advisory committee meetings are advised that the agency is not responsible for providing access to electrical outlets.

FDA welcomes the attendance of the public at its advisory committee meetings and will make every effort to accommodate persons with physical disabilities or special needs. If you require special accommodations due to a disability, please contact Trevelin Prysock at 301–827–7001 at least 7 days in advance of the meeting.

Notice of this meeting is given under the Federal Advisory Committee Act (5 U.S.C. app. 2).

Dated: November 9, 2004.

Sheila Dearybury Walcoff,
Associate Commissioner for External Relations.

[FR Doc. 04–25530 Filed 11–17–04; 8:45 am]

BILLING CODE 4160–01–S

DEPARTMENT OF HEALTH AND HUMAN SERVICES

National Institutes of Health

Office of the Director, National Institutes of Health; Notice of Meeting

Pursuant to section 10(d) of the Federal Advisory Committee Act, as amended (5 U.S.C. Appendix 2), notice is hereby given of the meeting of the Advisory Committee to the Director, National Institutes of Health (NIH).

The meeting will be open to the public as indicated below, with attendance limited to space available. Individuals who plan to attend and need special assistance, such as sign language interpretation or other reasonable accommodations, should notify the Contact Person listed below in advance of the meeting.

A portion of the meeting will be closed to the public in accordance with the provisions set forth in the Government in the Sunshine Act, sections 552b(c)(6) and 552b(c)(9)(B), Title 5 U.S.C., as amended, because the disclosure of which would constitute a clearly unwarranted invasion of personal property and the premature disclosure of information and the discussions are likely to significantly

A Subcommittee was established at the SACHRP's fourth meeting on October 5, 2004, to provide assistance in addressing issues related to the specified topics.

On February 1, 2005, SACHRP will hear presentations from experts on the following topics: Adverse Events reporting and Compliance Oversight Issues.

Public attendance at the meeting is limited to space available. Individuals who plan to attend the meeting and need special assistance, such as sign language interpretation or other reasonable accommodations, should notify the designated contact persons. Members of the public will have the opportunity to provide comments on both days of the meeting. Public comment will be limited to five minutes per speaker. Any members of the public who wish to have printed materials distributed to SACHRP members for this scheduled meeting should submit materials to the Executive Director, SACHRP, prior to the close of business on January 14, 2005.

Information about SACHRP and the draft meeting agenda will be posted on the SACHRP Web site at http://www.dhhs.gov/ohrp/sachrp/index.html.

Dated: December 10, 2004.

Bernard A. Schwetz,
Director, Office for Human Research Protections, Executive Secretary, Secretary's Advisory Committee on Human Research Protections.

[FR Doc. 04–27490 Filed 12–15–04; 8:45 am]
BILLING CODE 4150-36-P

DEPARTMENT OF HEALTH AND HUMAN SERVICES

Centers for Disease Control and Prevention

Disease, Disability, and Injury Prevention and Control Special Emphasis Panel (SEP): Reproductive Health Research, Request for Applications Number (RFA) DP–05–010

In accordance with Section 10(a)(2) of the Federal Advisory Committee Act (Public Law 92–463), the Centers for Disease Control and Prevention (CDC) announces the following meeting:

Name: Disease, Disability, and Injury Prevention and Control Special Emphasis Panel (SEP): Reproductive Health Research, RFA DP–05–010.

Times and Dates: 8:30 a.m.–9 a.m., January 10, 2005 Panel A (Open). 9 a.m.–5 p.m., January 10, 2005 Panel A (Closed). 9 a.m.–2 p.m., January 11, 2005 Panel A (Closed). 8:30 a.m.–9 a.m., January 11, 2005 Panel B (Open). 9 a.m.–5 p.m., January 11, 2005 Panel B (Closed). 9 a.m.–2 p.m., January 12, 2005 Panel B (Closed). 8:30 a.m.–9 a.m., January 12, 2005 Panel C (Open). 9 a.m.–5 p.m., January 12, 2005 Panel C (Closed). 9 a.m.–5 p.m., January 13, 2005 Panel C (Closed).

Place: Sheraton Colony Square Hotel, 188 14th Street, NE., Atlanta, GA 30361, Telephone Number 404.892.6000.

Status: Portions of the meeting will be closed to the public in accordance with provisions set forth in Section 552b(c) (4) and (6), Title 5 U.S.C., and the Determination of the Director, Management Analysis and Services Office, CDC, pursuant to Public Law 92–463.

Matters to be Discussed: The meeting will include the review, discussion, and evaluation of applications received in response to: Reproductive Health Research, RFA DP–05–010.

Contact Person for More Information: Antonia J. Spadaro, EdD, Centers for Disease Control and Prevention, National Center for Chronic Disease and Health Promotion, 4770 Buford Hwy, Mailstop K–92, Atlanta, GA 30341, Telephone 770.488.5809.

The Director, Management Analysis and Services Office, has been delegated the authority to sign **Federal Register** notices pertaining to announcements of meetings and other committee management activities, for both CDC and the Agency for Toxic Substances and Disease Registry.

Dated: December 8, 2004.

Alvin Hall,
Director, Management Analysis and Services Office, Centers for Disease Control and Prevention (CDC).

[FR Doc. 04–27516 Filed 12–15–04; 8:45 am]
BILLING CODE 4163-18-P

DEPARTMENT OF HEALTH AND HUMAN SERVICES

Centers for Disease Control and Prevention

Procedures and Costs for Use of the Research Data Center; Amendment

In the notice document announcing the "Procedures and Costs for Use of the Research Data Center," appearing on page 67584 in the **Federal Register** issue of Thursday, November 18, 2004, the notice is amended to extend the comment period as follows:

On page 67584 under the **DATES** heading, change "December 9, 2004", to "March 1, 2005."

All other information in the document remains unchanged.

Dated: December 8, 2004.

James D. Seligman,
Associate Director for Program Services, Centers for Disease Control and Prevention (CDC).

[FR Doc. 04–27514 Filed 12–15–04; 8:45 am]
BILLING CODE 4163-18-P

DEPARTMENT OF HEALTH AND HUMAN SERVICES

Centers for Medicare & Medicaid Services

Privacy Act of 1974; Report of Modified or Altered System

AGENCY: Department of Health and Human Services (HHS) Centers for Medicare & Medicaid Services (CMS).

ACTION: Notice of proposed modification or alteration to a system of records (SOR).

SUMMARY: In accordance with the requirements of the Privacy Act of 1974, we are proposing to modify or alter an SOR, "Unique Physician/Practitioner Identification Number (UPIN) (formerly known as the Medicare Physician Identification and Eligibility System)," System No. 09–70–0525. We propose to delete published routine use number 1 authorizing disclosure to contractors for refining or processing records, and in connection with Automated Data Processing software or a telecommunication system containing or supporting records in the system, number 3 authorizing disclosure to the Railroad Retirement Board (RRB), number 6 authorizing disclosure to the Department of Justice (DOJ) for investigating and prosecuting violations of the Social Security Act (the Act), number 7 authorizing disclosure to state licensing boards for review of unethical practices or non-professional conduct, and an unnumbered routine use authorizing disclosure to the Social Security Administration (SSA). Disclosures that were previously permitted under published routine use number 1 will now be authorized under proposed routine use number 2. Proposed routine use number 2 will release information to "agency contractors or consultants" who have been engaged by the agency to assist in accomplishment of a CMS function related to this system of records (SOR).

Disclosures previously permitted under published routine uses number 3, 7, and to the SSA will be authorized by proposed routine use number 3, which will release information to "another Federal and/or state agency, agency of a state government, an agency established by state law, or its fiscal agent."

Disclosures authorizing release to DOJ for investigating and prosecuting violations of the Act will be carried out under proposed routine use number 9, which authorizes release of data to "combat fraud and abuse." We propose to add 3 new routine uses to provide disclosure of records when all